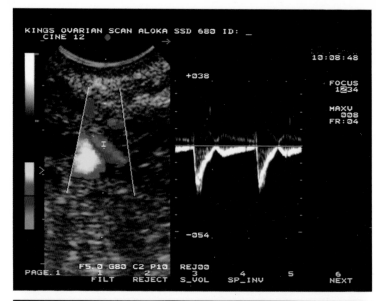

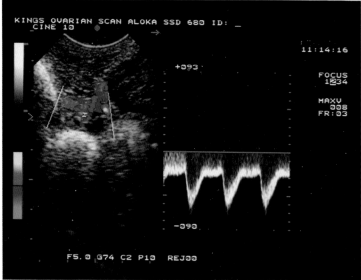

Flow velocity waveforms obtained from the uterine artery of a postmenopausal woman before (top figure) and after (bottom figure) 12 days of therapy with transdermal oestradiol 50 µg/day.

The position of the Doppler gate across the uterine artery is displayed on the left-hand side of both figures, and the flow velocity waveform display shown on the right-hand side. Changes over at least two cardiac cycles are demonstrated.

The pre-treatment waveform shows reduced flow during diastole with a 'notch' at the end of systole. This indicates increased impedance to flow distal to the point of sampling. Transdermal oestradiol 50 µg/day for 12 days increases end-diastolic flow and eliminates the notch. Thus, impedance to flow is reduced.

See pages 63 and 64 for further details. [Reproduced with permission of Bourne T, Hillard T and Whitehead MI: Menopause and Ovarian Scanning Clinics, King's College Hospital, 1991 (unpublished observations).]

Hormone Replacement Therapy
Your Questions Answered

By

Malcolm Whitehead FRCOG

Senior Lecturer/Honorary Consultant,
Academic Department of Obstetrics and Gynaecology,
King's College School of Medicine and Dentistry, London;
Medical Director, Amarant Trust, London, UK

Val Godfree MRCOG

Honorary Lecturer,
Academic Department of Obstetrics and Gynaecology,
King's College School of Medicine and Dentistry, London;
Deputy Medical Director, Amarant Trust, London, UK

Foreword by
David W. Purdie MD FRCOG FSA (Scot)

Professor,
Director of Postgraduate Education Centre,
Hull Royal Infirmary, Hull, UK

CHURCHILL LIVINGSTONE
EDINBURGH LONDON MADRID MELBOURNE NEW YORK AND TOKYO 1992

CHURCHILL LIVINGSTONE
Medical Division of Longman Group UK Limited

Distributed in the United States of America by Churchill
Livingstone Inc., 650 Avenue of the Americas, New York, N.Y.
10011, and by associated companies, branches and representatives
throughout the world.

© Longman Group UK Limited 1992

First edition 1992

ISBN 0-443-04353-1

British Library Cataloguing in Publication Data
A catalogue record for this book is available from the British Library

Library of Congress Cataloging in Publication Data available

Printed and bound in Great Britain by
Butler & Tanner Ltd, Frome and London

Foreword

For an event first described in the book of Genesis, the menopause has been a long time in the shadows of myth and superstition. It is only in recent decades that the spotlight of serious enquiry has been shone on an event which, given the longevity of our womenfolk, is almost literally central to their lives. For, with female life expectancy in the developed world approaching 80 years a woman may, on average, expect to spend some 30 years — or 40% of her active life — in the postmenopausal era.

The time of menopause is remarkably stable down the generations and indeed across the continents, this conservation marking it out as a feature which has proved to be of value to the success and survival of our species. Indeed, the menopause does confer advantage by terminating the possibility of late conception and freeing the mother to guide and protect her last offspring through the long human childhood.

The benefit to the species, however, may be less than obvious to the individual. The climacteric, that transition from fertility to infertility of which the menopause is a part, may be attended by symptoms whose severity and duration simply cannot be predicted. Equally, the longer term effects of the menopause on heart, bone and brain are now well appreciated. Hence the approach of this phase of a woman's life may be attended by rising apprehension and genuine fear, associated as it often is with the departure of children and the death of parents. The best antidote to fear is, as always, knowledge. It is every women's right to be advised — and in plain language — what the menopause is, what it brings in its train, and what may be done about it. It is the duty of all doctors who care for women to be available to them at this difficult time and to consider for hormone replacement those women likely to derive short or long-term benefit from it. However, not all women are seen by, or indeed wish to see, their doctors during the time of menopause and it is therefore essential that our accumulated knowledge is marshalled in an accessible form for them.

Malcolm Whitehead and Valerie Godfree have taken as their starting point in this book the very questions which real women ask of real doctors.

They then proceed to answer those questions in lucid English while embodying the most recent scientific insights into the subject. The result is a warm yet objective consultation in which every women of this age will recognize herself and as a result of which she can decide whether to consult her own doctor. Never before have so many women reached the menopause and never before have we known so much about the subject. It is timely, therefore, that both knowledge and women be brought together, as in this book, with the immediate aim of dispelling myth and the ultimate aim of promoting health and fulfilment in the years that lie ahead.

1991   D.W.P.

Preface

If we had written this book 15–20 years ago it would have been no more than 30 pages in length. It would have discussed the value of cyclical oestrogens, given 3 weeks out of every 4 (and unopposed by a progestogen), in relieving the acute symptoms of ovarian failure principally the hot flushes and night sweats. This volume runs to approximately 230 pages and the 'question and answer' format covers not only symptomatic and psychological changes associated with oestrogen lack and replacement, but also the relationships between oestrogens and progestogens with the principal other vulnerable end-organs that they affect, such as the breast, the endometrium, the arterial tree and bone status.

It is most probably because of this wide spectrum of activity that hormone replacement therapy (HRT) is so controversial. Few therapies are capable of potentially being so advantageous (reduction in risk of coronary artery disease and osteoporotic fracture) yet so disadvantageous (questionable increase in risk of breast cancer with long-term use). Because the profound effects of HRT on these diseases have only been appreciated relatively recently, sufficient time has not elapsed for the *precise* benefits and risks of different preparations and routes of administration to be fully elucidated, although an overall pattern has emerged. Furthermore, doctor and patient attitudes will be influenced by personal experience. For example, the women who has nursed her mother through terminal breast or endometrial cancer is likely to avoid HRT; her counterpart, who watched her mother die, perhaps prematurely, from a disease which HRT can protect against, such as hip fracture or myocardial infarction, may well request preventative therapy.

Personal biases must be put aside when population health is considered. Between the ages of 50 and 94 years, it has been estimated that a white women's cumulative absolute risk of cause-specific death from coronary artery disease is 31%; from breast cancer it is 2.8%, from hip fracture it is also 2.8%, and from endometrial cancer it is 0.7%. HRT, administered for 5-10 years soon after menopause, appears to reduce the risk of coronary artery disease by approximately 50%. If this benefit is maintained into later years then it will dwarf all other effects of oestrogens. It is for this reason that the benefits of HRT will greatly outweigh the potential disadvantages in population terms.

The aim of this book is to provide guidance about HRT to doctors and other healthcare specialists who see and counsel women about menopause-related problems. Patients who are familiar with medical terminology may also find it of value. The 'question and answer' format has been adopted so that it can be used for rapid reference. Although this book contains the most up-to-date thinking on the short- and long-term effects of HRT on responsive tissues, we have tried to emphasize clinical aspects which, we hope, will assist the physician in his or her day-to-day management. Thus, this book contains practical as well as theoretical information. In addition to researching and contributing to the literature, we supervise three Menopause Clinics in London (in the Academic Department of Obstetrics and Gynaecology at King's College Hospital, at Queen Charlotte's Maternity and the Chelsea Hospital for Women, and at the Amarant Centre at the Churchill Clinic) that, between them, perform approximately 16 000 appointments each year. This is a greater workload than the outpatient gynaecological services provided by most hospitals and our clinical approach has evolved from more than 20 years combined experience.

When planning this book, we anticipated that the average physician (if one exists!) would refer to individual sections or chapters, piecemeal. Although each chapter addresses one principal issue of the menopause or HRT and can stand alone, we have tried in each chapter to put that issue into a broad prospective. Thus, some repetition has occurred but we make no apology for this. We have not referenced the text but have included a 'Guide to further reading'. Controversial areas are clearly indicated as are those where too few data exist for reliable guidelines to be recommended.

We acknowledge the tremendous help of Mrs Angela Short who typed the entire manuscript: of Dr Timothy Hillard for contributing to Chapters 6 and 8, and of our Research Fellows, Drs Sovra Whitcroft, Michael Ellerington and Michael Marsh for help with the artwork and for proof-reading. We would also like to thank Ms Amanda Ryde and Ms Katia Chrysostomou at Churchill Livingstone for all their support and patience.

London,   M.W.
1991   V.G.

Contents

1. The menopause – a growing problem

The menopause is a physiological event that occurs in all women living beyond the age of 60 years. There is now little doubt that it can be associated with distressing symptoms and long-term life-threatening diseases such as osteoporosis and arterial disease. It is no longer appropriate to dismiss these problems as the inevitable consequences of ageing or that the only management required is sympathy and emotional support. Over the last 10–20 years enormous strides have been made in our understanding of both the short and long-term consequences of oestrogen deficiency, and the benefits of hormone replacement therapy (HRT) have been shown clearly to outweigh the risks.

1.1 Why is this termed a growing problem?

The problems of the climacteric have assumed a greater importance during the course of this century because there has been a striking increase in average female life expectancy. Thus many, many women are now living beyond the time of the menopause and into old age (Fig. 1.1). In 1850 the average female life expectancy was approximately 40 years; at the turn of the 20th century it had increased to approximately 55 years. At present, the average female life expectancy is approximately 80 years. Thus, women today can expect to live approximately 30 years in the postmenopausal, oestrogen-deficient state. Table 1.1 illustrates how women's life expectancy has increased over the last three decades and is expected to go on increasing.

There are almost 10 million women over the age of 50 in the UK at present and they comprise 17% of the total UK population. The latter is expected to peak around the year 2029. By this time there will be almost 12.5 million women over the age of 50 and they will comprise more than 20% of the total population. Women in the age group 45–59 years will increase in numbers by 20% over the course of the next decade, and 32% over the next 30 years. There will be corresponding increases in the older

1

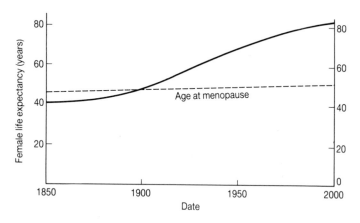

Fig. 1.1 Rise in female life expectancy in the last 150 years. (From Fraser D 1989 Horizons, July, 459. Reproduced with permission.)

Table 1.1 Female expectation of life in the UK

	Year		
Age	1955	1987	2027
0	73	78	81
15	60	64	66
50	27	30	32
60	19	21	23
65	15	17	19
75	9	11	12

From the Government Actuaries Department, Office of Population, Census and Surveys, Series PP2 no. 16.

age groups but in particular there will be a 50% increase in the number of women over the age of 85 years during the next 20–30 years (Fig. 1.2).

Thus, there has been an enormous increase in the number of postmenopausal women in our society over the course of this century which is going to continue over the next 30 years at least. Whilst the numerical increase in postmenopausal women is well documented it is more difficult to assess the change in aspirations that has occurred within this group. It is probably true that women today have greater expectations of a higher quality of life than previous generations. Therefore, it seems likely that climacteric and postmenopausal women will continue to place increasing demands on health care resources for many years to come.

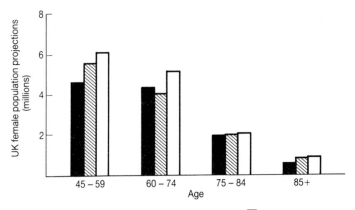

Fig. 1.2   UK female population over 45 years of age in 1987 (■) and projected changes in the years 2001 (▨) and 2021 (□). (From the Population Projections Series PP2 no. 16. Office of Population Census and Surveys.)

1.2 The age at menarche has decreased over the years; has there been a corresponding change in the average age at menopause?

No. It appears that average age at menopause has changed little over the centuries. In each period, classical, medieval, and modern, 50 years has remained the modal age. The primary difference between age at menopause in classical times and that of today's industrialized nations, is that women in ancient times did not usually live beyond fertility to menopause.

Studies have failed to establish that age at menopause has a specific relationship to the age at menarche. Many other specific variables have been studied for possible influence on age at menopause but relatively few have been demonstrated as statistically significant. Only two factors appear to play a significant role in the determination of age at menopause: altitude and cigarette smoking. High altitudes are found to accelerate menopausal age. Heavy smokers can expect to experience an earlier menopause than non-smokers. As yet, the oral contraceptive pill has not been studied for its short and long-term effects on age and/or experience of natural menopause.

1.3 What are the potential benefits of HRT?

A therapeutic role for HRT was clearly established many years ago. More recently its preventive role has been clarified. Thus, many doctors are now re-examining their policies towards climacteric and postmenopausal women. Studies have consistently shown that 3 out of every 4 women experience climacteric symptoms, to varying degrees. It is true that many of these women experiencing distressing symptoms have remained untreated in the past, despite seeking medical advice. Osteoporosis and arterial disease are significant causes of morbidity and mortality in postmenopausal women and therefore hormone replacement therapy can make a very significant contribution in improving the wellbeing of individuals and of society as a whole.

1.4 What, in simple terms, are the morbidity and mortality associated with osteoporotic fracture and arterial disease, and how does HRT affect them?

Forty to 50% of British women will experience an osteoporotic fracture before the age of 75 years; a woman's lifetime risk of a fractured neck of femur is 15%, i.e. 1 in 7. It has been estimated that 5–6 years of HRT commencing in the early postmenopausal years will reduce the risk of hip and vertebral fracture by 50%. The incidence of hip fracture has doubled over the last 30 years, and 35 000 women fractured a hip in 1985. The mortality rate from fractured neck of femur is between 17% and 20% and many of those who survive the fracture become permanently dependent on nursing care. Thus, it can be seen that osteoporosis is a serious disease but is now regarded as a preventable one. As yet, HRT is the treatment of choice for prevention of osteoporosis.

Arterial disease (cardiovascular and cerebrovascular disease) remains the largest single cause of death amongst women in this country. There is considerable epidemiological evidence that oestrogen replacement therapy reduces the mortality from cardiovascular disease by 50% and cerebrovascular disease by approximately 30–50%. Taking osteoporosis and arterial disease into account HRT has a significant preventive role both in terms of preventing morbidity and reducing mortality.

1.5 What are the major risks of HRT?

The risk of increasing endometrial cancer with unopposed oestrogen therapy has been eliminated with modern regimens which include adequate progestogen courses along with the oestrogen. One outstanding concern is that HRT will increase the risk of breast cancer. At present, data on short-term use of HRT (up to 5–6 years) are reassuring and many experts now accept that short-term use of HRT does not increase the risk of breast cancer significantly. However, long-term use of HRT (longer than 10 years) may involve an increase in risk of perhaps 10–45%. It is hoped that further studies will help to clarify this situation.

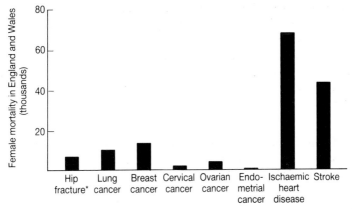

Fig. 1.3 Deaths in women of all ages in England and Wales by selected underlying causes in 1987. * Deaths from hip fractures are estimated. (From Mortality Statistics: cause. Series DH2 no. 14. Office of Population Census and Surveys, and Hospital In Patient Enquiry Series MB4 no. 29. Reproduced by permission.)

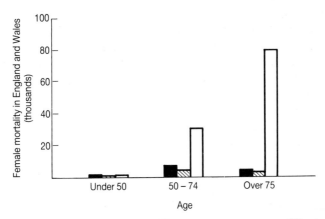

Fig. 1.4 Deaths in women from breast cancer (■), gynaecological malignancies (▨) and arterial disease (▢) according to age group, in England and Wales in 1987. Note: 'gynaecological malignancies includes adnexal neoplasms; arterial disease includes deaths from ischaemic heart disease and cerebrovascular disease. (From Mortality Statistics: cause. Series DH2 no. 14. Office of Population Census and Surveys.)

1.6 What is the relative importance of the major benefits and risks of HRT?

Figure 1.3 illustrates the most recent data on female mortality at all ages in England and Wales. It is clear that ischaemic heart disease and stroke are numerically far more important than breast cancer and all gynaecological malignancies combined. It is interesting to note that death from lung cancer has increased relatively rapidly, and this probably reflects the increase in cigarette smoking amongst the female population.

Figure 1.4 shows the relative importance of breast cancer, all gynaecological malignancies and all arterial disease as a cause of death in women aged under 50 years. Here, death from breast cancer outnumbers deaths from ischaemic heart disease and stroke combined. However, this pattern is reversed in the postmenopausal age groups in whom arterial disease death greatly exceeds death from breast cancer. The vast majority of HRT-users will belong to the groups aged over 50 years. However, breast cancer remains an important concern amongst both doctors and their patients. It is important that we put this fear into perspective when trying to make an assessment of the benefits and risks of HRT for each individual. The lifetime risk of a heart attack or stroke or hip fracture is greater than the lifetime risk of breast cancer. The benefits of HRT in terms of symptom relief and prevention of osteoporosis and arterial disease do appear to outweigh the possible risks and the disadvantages of therapy. However, the decision to initiate and continue with therapy is one that must be taken jointly between the doctor and patient. As doctors it is our duty to ensure that our patients have an opportunity to make an informed choice.

2. The climacteric: definitions and endocrinology

2.1 What is meant by the terms menopause and climacteric?

The menopause is defined as the last menstrual period. The climacteric is the transitional phase during which ovarian function ceases and which, when complete, leads to the postmenopause. The terms are used interchangeably but strictly speaking they should not be. The climacteric is sometimes called the perimenopause.

2.2 When do they occur?

The median age of menopause is 50.8 years and has changed but little during this century. It appears to be unaffected by socio-economic conditions, race, parity, height, weight or skin fold thickness. However, tobacco users appear to undergo a natural menopause 1–2 years earlier than non-smokers.

The age at which menopause occurs varies greatly. Our youngest patient who is truly postmenopausal (i.e. ovarian failure due to loss of oocytes) is 18 years old: conversely, we also not infrequently see women who have not undergone menopause until age 58–59 years.

For most women the climacteric extends for 2–3 years, and usually starts around age 46–48 years. However, in some women the climacteric may last very much longer with the initial symptoms of ovarian failure starting in the late 30s/early 40s and predating menopause by 8–10 years.

2.3 Why do the climacteric and menopause occur?

Oestradiol production can be considered a by-product of oocyte maturation: progesterone production by the ovary only occurs after ovulation. A reduction in ovarian responsiveness to gonadotrophin stimulation, together with depletion and finally exhaustion of oocytes, results in a gradual decline in oestradiol production. When anovulation becomes more frequent there is a loss of progesterone production by the ovary. Eventually, oestradiol production falls below a critical threshold and endometrial stimulation no longer occurs. Amenorrhoea results.

2.4 What are the endocrine changes associated with the climacteric?

1. The initiating event is ovarian unresponsiveness to gonadotrophic stimulation. The precise cause is unclear but involves oocyte depletion, and perhaps loss of inhibin production together with changes in the circulating forms of the principal gonadotrophins, follicle stimulating hormone (FSH) and luteinizing hormone (LH). One consequence of the ovarian unresponsiveness is that FSH levels rise and initially this is a cyclical phenomenon. The length of the menstrual cycle shortens, usually from about 28 to 21−24 days. This is primarily due to a reduction in the follicular phase of the menstrual cycle.

2. As ovarian unresponsiveness becomes more marked, the length of the menstrual cycle may increase to any duration between 28 days and many months.

3. Eventually most cycles are anovulatory. Corpus luteum function is deficient and progesterone production falls markedly. Oestradiol secretion may be erratic and the length of the anovulatory cycle can range from as short as 14 days to as long as many months.

4. Complete failure of follicular development results in a further reduction in plasma oestradiol levels. Eventually, they fall below a critical threshold and endometrial proliferation ceases. Amenorrhoea then ensues. The menopause is the last menstrual period and it is the only constant feature of the climacteric.

5. Increased gonadotrophin secretion, to drive the failing ovary, occurs throughout the latter stages of the climacteric and plasma gonadotrophin levels are elevated. These may reach a maximum 2−3 years after menopause and then decline gradually during the next 20−30 years. As compared to premenopausal values, FSH levels may increase 18-fold and LH levels by a factor of 3. These changes are illustrated in Figure 2.1.

6. The contribution made by the postmenopausal ovary to the circulating sex hormone pool in plasma is controversial. Some authors have reported that the postmenopausal ovary makes little useful contribution, but others argue that it contributes small but biologically active amounts of various

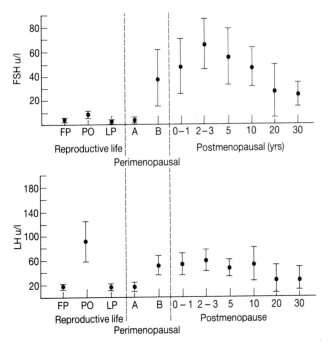

Fig. 2.1 Mean (± 1SD) plasma FSH and LH values in pre-, peri- and postmenopausal women. FP = follicular phase, PO = peak ovulatory value, LP = luteal phase. A and B are women still menstruating with apparent menopausal symptoms. B are women complaining of vasomotor symptoms. [Adapted from Studd J W W, Chakravarti S, Oram D 1977. In Greenblatt R, Studd J W W (eds) Clinics in Obstetrics and Gynecology. W B Saunders, London and Philadelphia 4(1): p 6. Reproduced with permission].

hormones, particularly androstenedione and testosterone. The adrenal gland continues to produce both the latter hormones after menopause. Irrespective of whether significant ovarian function continues after menopause or not, there can be no doubt that as compared to the premenopausal era, the postmenopause is associated with a relative excess of androgens to oestrogens. This may explain why so many postmenopausal women complain of unwanted hair growth; and why lipid and lipoprotein metabolism undergoes profound changes which may influence the later risk of certain arterial diseases.

In the postmenopausal woman, the predominant circulating oestrogen is oestrone. The source is peripheral conversion of androstenedione, currently believed to take place largely in adipose tissue, to oestrone. Although plasma oestrone values are lower in postmenopausal women than during the reproductive era, the fall in plasma oestradiol values from pre- to

Table 2.1 Principal hormone changes following loss of ovarian function

Hormone	Change	Comment
Oestradiol (E2)	↓↓↓	Principal postmenopausal source of oestradiol appears to be peripheral conversion from oestrone; controversy exists over small ovarian source
Oestrone (E1)	↓↓	Principal circulating oestrogen postmenopause. Derived from conversion of androgens
Ratio E1:E2	↑	Reversal of premenopausal ratio
FSH	↑↑↑	
LH	↑	
Androstenedione	↓	Reduction after natural menopause but small as compared to fall in oestradiol. Most authors report lower plasma values after castration
Testosterone	↓	
Ratio androgen:oestrogen	↑	Relative androgen excess after menopause as compared to premenopausal values

Table 2.2 Serum sex steriod concentration before and after natural or surgical menopause

	Oestrone (E1) pmol/l	Oestradiol (E2) pmol/l	Progesterone nmol/l	Testosterone nmol/l	Androstenedione nmol/l
Premenopausal					
Early follicular	90–180	90–350	0.3–1.6	0.7–1.4	5.6–6.1
Late follicular	550–740	740–1390	–	1.0–2.8	6.4–7.0
Mid luteal	260–370	520–870	>20–30	1.0–2.1	–
Postmenopausal					
Natural	75–150	35–55	0.3–0.8	0.7–1.0	2.1–3.1
Surgical	75–150	35–55	0.3–0.8	0.3–0.6	1.7–2.8

postmenopause is much greater. Thus, the relative predominance of oestradiol over oestrone seen during the reproductive era is reversed in the postmenopause.

The principal hormone changes that occur during the climacteric and into the postmenopause are outlined in Table 2.1; the plasma concentrations of the more important steroid hormones, pre- and postmenopausally, are presented in Table 2.2.

2.5 What changes in the menstrual cycle can be expected during the climacteric?

1. Early during the climacteric, the menstrual cycle may shorten to 21 – 24 days but the menstrual loss usually remains normal. Occasionally, women may 'miss' a period for one or perhaps two cycles. These episodes tend to be associated with flushes and sweats. The vasomotor symptoms resolve when ovarian function returns, manifest as a resumption of menstruation.

2. Later on, the cycle may lengthen to any duration between 28 days and many months but it may still be ovulatory. The menstrual loss may be normal or scantier.

3. Anovulatory cycles can be quite unpredictable, ranging in length from 14 days to many months. The duration of bleeding is also variable; it may last for only a few hours or may be heavy and last for many days (metropathia haemorrhagica).

4. Rarely, the menstrual cycle may be quite regular until menstruation ceases abruptly.

5. The timescale over which these changes may occur is extremely variable and may differ greatly from one individual to another.

2.6 Is the postmenopausal woman totally oestrogen deficient?

No. The peripheral conversion of androstenedione to oestrone has already been referred to. Because this occurs largely in fat, obese women tend to produce more oestrone than their thin counterparts. Oestrone, on a weight-for-weight basis, is less biologically active than oestradiol but it still possesses the ability to bind to the oestradiol receptor and cause oestrogenic effects within responsive cells. Furthermore, small amounts of oestrone may undergo further conversion to oestradiol. Obese postmenopausal women are said to suffer less than thin women from oestrogen-deficiency symptoms such as hot flushes and night sweats, but data to support this statement are difficult to find. In general terms, obese women are less likely to develop osteoporosis (however, this is not unknown), but are at an increased risk of endometrial cancer as compared to thin women. This most probably reflects their greater oestrogenic milieu.

3. Consequences of oestrogen deficiency

While there is no universally agreed classification of the effects of oestrogen deficiency, we find it makes most sense to classify them by their time of onset. Thus, the symptoms/consequences can be acute, intermediate or long-term and are illustrated in Table 3.1.

ACUTE SYMPTOMS

The acute symptoms often arise early during the climacteric when menstruation, albeit erratic, is still occurring. Although they are self-limiting in the majority of women, a minority continue to experience these symptoms for many years. The ability of these symptoms to reduce the quality of life is poorly defined, but appears to be considerable in some women. Their effects in the workplace have still to be determined.

3.1 What are the acute symptoms of the climacteric?

The acute symptoms are the vasomotor disturbances together with the psychological problems. It is likely that they are interdependent to some extent, and they may share a common neuroendocrine aetiology.

3.2 Why do they arise?

The precise pathophysiology of vasomotor symptoms is not known. The occurrence of flushes and sweats is not related to the *absolute* plasma oestrogen concentrations, but their onset may be related to the rate of change in the plasma concentrations.

Preliminary results have suggested that the occurrence of flushing and sweating episodes is related to the 'free' plasma oestradiol level (that part of the oestradiol pool not bound in plasma to sex hormone binding globulin). Confirmatory data are awaited.

The onset of individual flushing and sweating episodes is related to a discharge of LH from the pituitary. However, abolition of the LH surge does not affect the frequency nor the severity of flushing and sweating

Table 3.1 Acute, intermediate and long-term symptoms associated with oestrogen deficiency

Symptoms/Disease	System	Time onset
Hot flushes Night Sweats Insomnia	Vasomotor	Acute
		months
Mood changes Anxiety Irritability Poor memory Poor concentration Loss of self-esteem	Neuroendocrine	Menstruation ceases
Genital tract atrophy Dyspareunia Urethral syndrome Loss of libido	Lower urogenital tract	months
Skin thinning ?Joint aches and pains ?Prolapse ?Incontinence	Connective tissue	
Cerebrovascular accident Coronory heart disease	Arterial	years
Osteoporosis	Skeletal	Chronic

episodes. Therefore, the LH surges are not causal. The current belief is that the disturbance responsible for flushing and sweating episodes arises somewhere within the hypothalamus. It has been proposed that there is an imbalance between certain neuro-transmitters, particularly the catecholamines (adrenaline, noradrenaline) and the catechol oestrogens, and that this imbalance occurs somewhere near the thermo-regulatory centre.

Oestrogen deficiency may result in lower levels of the catechol oestrogens within the CNS, and the effects of catecholamines on this centre are then not opposed adequately.

Oestradiol receptors have been located in most parts of the CNS in lower mammals. Psychological problems which increase in frequency during the climacteric (anxiety, irritability) may be a result of loss of oestradiol. Alternatively, these problems may be due, at least in part, to chronic sleep deprivation secondary to frequent night sweats. We suspect that both mechanisms operate.

3.3 What are vasomotor symptoms and when do they occur?
The commonest acute vasomotor symptoms are hot flushes and night sweats. The latter often result in insomnia. They are sometimes

accompanied by fainting episodes, palpitation and headaches, and they may arise early in the climacteric when menstruation is still regular. At this time, these symptoms tend to cluster in the premenstrual week and may then be confused with premenstrual syndrome (PMS). However, vasomotor symptoms can begin later, around the time of the menopause, or they may not develop until early during the postmenopausal years.

3.4 How many women suffer and to what degree?

Approximately 75% of climacteric and early postmenopausal women experience vasomotor symptoms. One third of these suffer acute physical distress as well as embarrassment. It is not known why approximately 25% of women do not have these symptoms.

3.5 As far as vasomotor symptoms are concerned, is there any difference between a natural and surgical menopause?

A surgical or radiotherapy-induced menopause is associated with a higher incidence and with an increased severity of vasomotor symptoms. The reasons for this are not clear. However, it has been suggested that the climacteric allows women to adjust gradually to lower circulating oestradiol concentrations, and that those who acclimatise best have fewer hot flushes and night sweats. An abrupt menopause does not allow for a period of gradual readjustment to the lower plasma levels and, therefore, these symptoms arise abruptly and are more severe.

3.6 How long do vasomotor symptoms last?

70% of symptomatic women have vasomotor symptoms for 2 years; 25% have vasomotor symptoms for 5 years and 5% have vasomotor symptoms ad infinitum.

3.7 What are hot flushes?

Women usually describe the flushes as unpleasant sensations of heat beginning in the face, neck, head or chest and spreading in any direction, sometimes over the whole body. Often the face becomes reddened and sweat may appear on the face, neck and trunk. Some women experience palpitation, dizziness or fainting with the flushing episode.

3.8 How often do hot flushes occur?

There is considerable individual variation in the frequency of hot flushes, ranging from a few per month to several per hour. Flushing may be episodic in character with quite marked symptoms lasting for several weeks followed by a relatively asymptomatic spell.

3.9 How long does a hot flush last?

Again, there is considerable individual variation in the duration of hot flushes, ranging from a few seconds to up to an hour with a mean around 3 minutes.

3.10 Are hot flushes always associated with sweating?

No. Some women rarely complain of sweating while others experience profuse sweating following intense flushing episodes. Some women complain of sweating with no prior flushing.

3.11 How troublesome are night sweats?

There is considerable variation in the frequency and the severity of night sweats. Some women find them very troublesome because sweating necessitates getting out of bed several times during the night to open a window, to take a shower, to change their clothing or occasionally to change the bed linen. This scenario can occur nightly over many weeks, months and sometimes years. It is a potent cause of sleep deprivation, not only to the woman but also to her partner.

3.12 Are there any environmental factors influencing hot flushes?

Sometimes flushes may be triggered by anxiety, hot weather, a change from a colder to a warmer environment, eating hot, spicy foods, or drinking hot drinks or alcohol. Most flushes, however, occur without an identifiable cause.

3.13 What is the association with sleep?

Sleep studies in climacteric women have shown that nocturnal flushing and sweating episodes are associated with periods of wakefulness, i.e. normal sleep rhythms are disrupted. It is interesting to note that while EEG recordings have detected episodes of waking, the subjects did not always remember the waking episodes in the morning.

3.14 What physiological changes occur during flushing episodes?

As stated previously, the precise physiological mechanism initiating hot flushes is unknown. Studies have shown that the subjective sensation

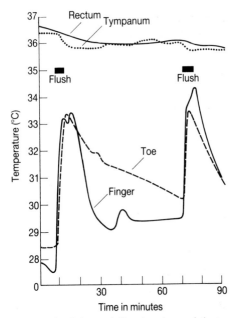

Fig. 3.1 Changes in peripheral (toe and finger) and central (rectum and timpanum) temperatures during two episodes of flushing in a postmenopausal woman. ■ = hot flush. (Adapted from Molnar G W 1975 Journal of Applied Physiology 38: 499–503. Reproduced with permission.)

of a flush precedes an initial increase in skin conductance (indicative of sweating) which is followed by vasodilatation with a rise in peripheral skin temperature of up to 5°C and fall in core body temperature of up to 1°C. The temperature changes are illustrated in Figure 3.1. These changes are associated with marked increases in heart rate of up to 20 beats per minute, fluctuations in baseline ECG recordings, abrupt increases in plasma adrenaline and decreases in noradrenaline, and the release of LH. Subsequently, skin conductance and sweating return to normal after about 20 minutes, while cutaneous vasodilatation and the rise in skin temperature may last as long as 40 minutes. It appears that the subjective sensation of heat is out of proportion to the actual rise in skin temperature. In addition, the temperature increase often persists for many minutes after the sensation of warmth has passed, indicating that the flush is only experienced while the skin temperature is rising.

3.15 Are hot flushes harmful?

No. But, many women find them embarrassing and this may affect their ability to cope at work and at home due to the avoidance of social contacts.

This may result in loss of self-confidence and of self-esteem. In addition, the importance of disturbed sleep patterns on a woman's general wellbeing should not be underestimated.

3.16 Can hormone profiles predict the severity of hot flushes?

No. There is no difference in the oestrogen level of postmenopausal women who have vasomotor symptoms and those who do not. However, some studies have identified a greater diurnal variation of plasma oestradiol in flushing women which suggests that the rate of change of the plasma oestrogen levels could be a trigger for the flushing mechanism, or that for each individual there is a range of oestrogen levels within which flushes will occur but above or below which they will not. This may explain why, eventually, most women cease having flushing and sweating episodes. Their plasma oestradiol values eventually fall below the critical range. We emphasize that this is speculation.

3.17 Both men and young girls have low oestrogen levels, why don't they have flushes?

The reason is still unclear since the precise role that oestrogens play in the causation of flushing remains to be established. However, it seems likely that priming with oestrogen is an essential prerequisite for flushing, i.e. an oestrogen milieu has to have been present and then withdrawn before flushing will occur. Women with ovarian dysgenesis do not have hot flushes unless they are given oestrogen replacement therapy which is later discontinued.

3.18 Are there any other conditions in which flushing and/or sweating occurs?

Yes. Other conditions associated with flushing and sweating are phaeo-chromocytoma, thyrotoxicosis and carcinoid syndrome but these cause additional symptoms which should make the true diagnosis obvious. Sweating can form part of a generalized anxiety disorder but the sweating of anxiety often affects other parts of the body such as the palms of the hands and soles of the feet, the flushing reaction does not occur and there is no nocturnal feature.

3.19 Can vasomotor symptoms cause psychological complaints?

Yes. Vasomotor instability can lead to chronic sleep deprivation and fatigue which may result in irritability, mood swings, indecisiveness and difficulties

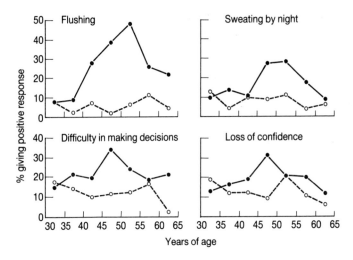

Fig. 3.2 Percentage of men (○-----○) and women (●——●) reporting the presence of various symptoms from age 30 years to age 65 years. (From Bungay G T, Vessey M P, McPherson C K 1980 British Medical Journal 2: 181–183. Reproduced with permission.)

with concentration. This is the so-called 'domino theory', i.e. psychological complaints are secondary manifestations of disabling vasomotor symptoms.

There is good evidence to show that the relief of vasomotor symptoms with oestrogen therapy has beneficial effects on the psychological status. See Question 4.7.

3.20 What are the psychological symptoms associated with the climacteric?

This remains a controversial area since evidence has been gathered by investigators from different scientific disciplines who have investigated different end-points. Many of the early studies were criticized because of methodological flaws.

More recent and better conducted studies have attempted to overcome these problems. Peaks of prevalence of flushing and sweating, difficulty in making decisions and loss of confidence have been shown to be closely associated with the climacteric (Fig. 3.2). Similar temporal responses have been obtained for anxiety, forgetfulness, difficulty in concentration and feelings of unworthiness. These psychological problems reach a peak prevalence immediately prior to the mean age of menopause. 'Depressed mood' has been reported as being significantly increased in peri- and postmenopausal women as compared with those still menstruating regularly. As might be predicted, vasomotor symptoms, sexual problems and sleep difficulties increase significantly from pre- to peri- to post-menopausal.

Twenty-five to 50% of women suffer some sort of psychological complaint during the climacteric years.

3.21 Why is there no consensus?

The controversy over the role a woman's hormones have on the psyche and on whether the hormonal changes at the climacteric are responsible for the various psychological symptoms described at this time has arisen for three main reasons. Firstly, studies have been performed on different groups of women; secondly, bias has been introduced in the epidemiological methods and thirdly the results have, on occasions, been misinterpreted.

Some investigators have recruited their study samples from menopause clinic populations while others are general population studies. While data on the nature and incidence rates of symptoms reported to clinicians at menopause clinics are valuable, they should be interpreted as applying only to selected groups of women and should not be applied to unselected groups of women within the community who for the most part experience less severe symptoms. Thus, it is not surprising that comparisons between such studies reveal inconsistencies and contraindications.

Many of the studies mention only chronological age and fail to define adequately endocrine or menopausal status. Almost all of the studies have been cross-sectional rather than longitudinal in design, and this fails to take into account the cohort differences which should be considered when comparing subjects across wide age ranges. There has been no standardized classification of psychological or somatic symptoms in these studies, and therefore comparisons are difficult. Few investigators have attempted to hide their interest in the climacteric and postmenopausal era and thus bias may have been introduced into responses. Finally, few studies have taken into account that the endocrine changes occur over a long period of time.

3.22 What other factors may contribute to psychological complaints?

Many clinicians accept that endocrine changes have a role in the generation of psychological complaints during the climacteric, but believe that these endocrine changes interact with socio-cultural factors, psychological factors (such as attitudes, expectations and personality) and stressful life events.

A detailed history is important in the management of climacteric women. However, it is sometimes difficult to make a precise assessment as to the cause of psychological complaints.

3.23 What social factors are important?

The climacteric has been viewed as a time of psycho-social stress involving role changes and life events such as bereavement, divorce or the departure of children from home. There is some evidence to suggest that bereavement, divorce or marital separation produces psychological and somatic symptoms but the departure of children from the home (the so-called 'empty nest syndrome') is not necessarily stressful. There are conflicting data as to whether adverse life events are more common perimenopausally. Whether these events are viewed as stressful or not may depend on a woman's attitude, personality and her general social situation. Lack of social supports, such as satisfactory relationships with a partner, family or friends, or the lack of available alternative roles such as employment may lead to greater symptom experience.

Other social factors such as social class, and marital and employment status have been considered in relation to psychological symptoms. Some studies have reported an increase in psychological and somatic symptoms in women of lower social class. Financial and housing difficulties may also be important. Studies investigating the association between psychological symptoms and marital or employment status have yielded conflicting results.

3.24 Are there any cultural differences in women's experience of the menopause?

There is some evidence to suggest that cultural factors may be important in determining a woman's response to the climacteric. For example, some studies in India and Africa and in some Arabian cultures have shown that women report few symptoms other than that of menstrual cycle change. These women eagerly awaited the menopause, since, in their culture, menopause is not viewed negatively and is not seen as a crisis.

3.25 What psychological factors may be important?

Factors such as attitude to the menopause, past experiences and personality will influence reactions to the menopause.

Women with negative attitudes to the menopause and with the expectation of difficulties are more likely to complain of psychological symptoms. In Western societies, menopausal woman is frequently given a negative stereotype, whether the menopause is associated with ageing and the loss of socially desirable characteristics such as youth and beauty or not.

There is some evidence that psychological symptoms are more prevalent in climacteric women with neurotic personality traits, current difficulties in coping with stresses and in those with low self-esteem.

3.26 Do those with a psychiatric history experience more problems at the menopause?

Perimenopausal women with a past history of psychiatric disorders report more psychological symptoms at the time of the menopause. One report has suggested that psychiatric disorder may lead to increased vasomotor symptoms.

3.27 Is there any increase in psychiatric disorders in perimenopausal women?

There is conflicting evidence as to whether the menopause is associated with an increased risk of psychiatric disorder or admission to hospital for a psychiatric illness.

3.28 Does the menopause cause depression?

The symptom of 'depressed mood' is often reported by perimenopausal women, and when combined with other symptoms such as feelings of worthlessness, anxiety, crying, fatigue, loss of drive, aches and pains, headaches, etc., it is easy to see why the clinical picture presented by some menopausal women is suggestive of clinical depression. While the classification of depressive illness remains controversial, the classical endogenous disorder is usually characterized by abnormal, persistent depressed mood associated with feelings of hopelessness, crying, suicidal tendencies, psychomotor retardation, impaired capacity to perform every-day social functions and other complaints suggesting physical illness such as appetite disturbance and weight loss. In most cases the problems presented by perimenopausal women are less severe and not continuous but fluctuating. Therefore, their depression is a symptom and rarely part of a true affective disorder.

3.29 How can oestrogen deficiency cause psychological symptoms?

Oestrogen deficiency may act in two ways:

1. In the 'domino theory', recurrent night sweats lead to chronic sleep deprivation which results in tiredness, fatigue and irritability, etc.

2. There is now some evidence that oestrogen deficiency has a direct effect on the CNS. Psychological complaints may reflect a change in CNS function secondary to changes in levels of certain steroids. Alternatively, symptoms could reflect an imbalance elsewhere. Catecholamine metabolism may be affected by endogenous and exogenous oestrogens and it is thought that altered catecholamine metabolism may be responsible for affective disorders.

Oestrogen receptors have been identified in the brain and appear to be concentrated in these areas currently believed to be associated with emotion. There is now good evidence for a 'mental tonic' effect of oestrogen. See Question 4.7.

INTERMEDIATE SYMPTOMS

3.30 What are the intermediate symptoms?

Intermediate symptoms can be classified into two main groups:
1. Those associated with atrophy of the lower urogenital tract.
2. Those associated with loss of collagen from connective tissue.

3.31 How many women are affected and when?

Intermediate symptoms are not self-limiting and tend to increase in frequency with time since menopause. Thus, 10–20% of our patients complain of some symptoms due to lower genital tract atrophy within 3 years of menopause, but this increases to 40–50% within 5–8 years of menopause. It is probable that the majority of women will have experienced at least one problem resulting from lower genital tract atrophy by 15–20 years after menopause.

The proportion of women developing symptoms due to collagen lack is undetermined at present.

3.32 What are the atrophic symptoms?

Oestrogen deficiency may result in atrophy of both the vagina and distal urethra since these tissues share a common embryological origin. Symptoms of atrophic vaginitis include vaginal dryness, dyspareunia and recurrent bacterial infections. Atrophy of the distal urethra may lead to the 'urethral syndrome', i.e. recurrent episodes of urinary frequency, dysuria and urgency.

3.33 What are the effects of oestrogen deficiency on the vagina?

The vaginal epithelium becomes thinner and there is some loss of vascularity and elasticity. The glycogen content of the epithelial, lining cells is reduced; therefore, the lactobacillus population is diminished and the pH increases. This reduces the resistance of the vagina to pyogenic organisms. Maturation of the vaginal epithelium is disturbed. Fewer mature superficial cells are produced and the proportion of immature parabasal cells increases.

The cumulative effect of these changes is of an increased predisposition to bacterial infection, and to a loss of vaginal secretions which some women are aware of all the time but many others notice most with intercourse. Finally, the vagina tends to become shorter, narrower and loses its characteristic rugae.

3.34 Do these changes affect libido?

Oestrogen deficiency can contribute to loss of libido after the menopause. A vicious circle can arise whereby oestrogen deficiency leads to vaginal dryness causing dyspareunia which, in turn, leads to less interest in sex, then less intercourse and even greater atrophy and more discomfort. Treatment of the oestrogen deficiency state can break this circle. See Question 4.10.

3.35 What are the effects of oestrogen deficiency on the bladder and urethra?

Conclusive data on a causal relationship between oestrogen deficiency and urinary tract dysfunction are lacking. However, there is evidence that the epithelium of the distal urethra is oestrogen dependent, and there is a correlation between symptoms of the urethral syndrome and changes in urethral cytology in postmenopausal women. Oestrogen therapy can exert beneficial effects on both symptoms and cytology. The relationship between oestrogens and function of the trigone is poorly defined. Preliminary data suggest that oestrogens may also act on the submucosal vascular plexuses and on the connective tissue layer of the urethra. The latter is rich in collagen fibres. There is an urgent need for more research into the precise impact of oestrogen deficiency on urinary function.

3.36 What symptoms can be attributed to an oestrogen-dependent loss of collagen?

The association between the oestrogen status and the collagen content of various structures is poorly defined at present. It is recognized that oestrogen deficiency causes a loss of collagen from the skin which results in skin thinning. Loss of collagen from around the urethra and within the trigone of the bladder may predispose to urinary dysfunction. The musculo-skeletal aches and pains of which many postmenopausal women complain may be related to a loss of collagen from ligaments and other soft tissues.

3.37 What are the effects of oestrogen deficiency on the skin?

A protein associated to the oestradiol receptor has been found in the superficial layers of the skin, in hair follicles and in sebaceous ducts.

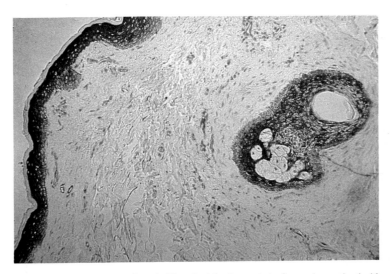

Fig. 3.3 Transverse section through skin stained for the presence of a protein associated with the oestradiol receptor; the dense staining shows the presence of the receptor in the epidermis, hair follicles and sebaceous ducts. [From Padwick M L, Whitehead M I, Coffer A, King R J B 1988 In: Studd J W W, Whitehead M I (eds) The Menopause. Blackwell Scientific, Oxford pp 227–233. Reproduced with permission.]

This is illustrated in Figure 3.3. This may account for the dry skin experienced by many postmenopausal women which improves with oestrogen replacement therapy.

There is a loss of collagen (a major constituent of the dermis) after the menopause. Skin collagen is lost at a faster rate during the immediate postmenopausal years than in the later years. Approximately 30% of collagen is lost during the first 5 years after menopause.

Complaints of thinning and dryness of the skin can be accompanied by increased bruising and itching. Very occasionally, 'crawling' sensations are experienced just underneath or on top of the skin. Women complain that they feel that 'ants are crawling over them'. This appears to represent a type of formication and is due, most likely, to changes in the peripheral nervous system rather than the result of changes in the skin, per se.

3.38 What other tissues are affected by oestrogen deficiency?

Other oestrogen target organs include the breast, uterus, fallopian tubes, ovaries, vagina and vulva as well as the urethra. Atrophic changes in oestrogen-dependent tissues is the rule after menopause although the frequency of symptoms varies greatly.

Following menopause, the vulva gradually undergoes atrophy with progressive loss of pubic hair and the skin becomes thinner. The subcutaneous tissues all but disappear and the labia shrink. The latter may contribute to dyspareunia. Although vulval dystrophies are more common in postmenopausal women, their relationship to oestrogen is poorly understood and vulval dystrophy is not considered a typical oestrogen deficiency consequence.

During the postmenopause, the uterus becomes smaller and the walls become thinner. The cervix is reduced in size. The endometrium becomes thin but, importantly, always retains the ability to respond to oestrogenic stimulation.

The tissues of the pelvic floor appear to lose tone and this may contribute to prolapse.

Certain other membranes also appear to be sensitive to ovarian function. For example, dryness of the mouth and eyes has been described as a menopausal disorder.

Breast involution follows loss of ovarian function. There is a reduction in the amount of glandular tissue with an increase in fat deposition and a relative predominance of connective tissue. However, involution is by no means a uniform process and there is great variation in the degree of atrophy observed in different parts of the breast and between individuals. The relative importance of oestrogen, progestogen and other hormones in this process is, as yet, uncertain.

LONG-TERM SEQUELAE

Whereas the acute and intermediate symptoms are not major causes of mortality, there can be no doubt that the two major long-term consequences of ovarian failure, osteoporosis and arterial disease, account for many deaths and are an important drain on financial resources. These sequelae do not usually arise until many years after ovarian failure and are clinically silent in the intervening period.

3.39 What are the long-term consequences of oestrogen deficiency?

The long-term problems caused by ovarian failure are osteoporosis and arterial disease.

3.40 Are women with acute symptoms at greater risk of these problems?

No. There is no evidence of a correlation between the presence or severity of vasomotor symptoms and the degree of later risk from osteoporosis or arterial disease. All postmenopausal women should be regarded as being potentially at risk from the long-term consequences of ovarian failure. We believe that it is important that all women should be made aware of these long-term consequences and that any attempt at population screening through Well Woman Clinics or health promotion clinics should include a full discussion of these issues.

Women undergoing premature menopause, whether natural or surgically induced, are more at risk from osteoporosis and arterial disease and therefore constitute a high-risk group. Every effort should be made to offer this group appropriate advice.

3.41 What is osteoporosis?

Osteoporosis can be defined as a reduction in bone density per unit volume which is sufficient to compromise the skeleton so that fracture may occur with minimal trauma. Thus, osteoporosis can be considered as loss of the 'engineering' strength of bone. There are many causes of osteoporosis. Age-related osteoporosis affects the majority of older men and women and is due to a decline in new bone formation. Postmenopausal osteoporosis, which is the type of osteoporosis considered here, is due to an increase in bone resorption and is the commonest metabolic bone disease in Western countries.

3.42 What are its effects?

Postmenopausal osteoporosis predisposes to fracture at certain skeletal sites. The most well recognized are the distal radius, the vertebrae and the proximal femur; less well recognized are the rib and the humerus.

3.43 Can established osteoporosis be treated?

Treatment of established bone loss is difficult because no currently available treatment modality will restore reduced bone density to normal. Therefore, prevention becomes all important.

3.44 Why is it considered important?

Postmenopausal osteoporosis is a serious, yet preventable, clinical problem affecting large numbers of women and resulting in significant morbidity, mortality and financial costs.

By around age of 80 years (which is the mean female life expectancy), approximately 40–50% of women will have developed osteoporosis and will have sustained at least one fracture. By age 80 years, one woman in eight will have sustained a hip fracture.

3.45 Does osteoporosis affect men too?

As indicated previously, there is an age-related loss of bone in both sexes. However, women have a lower bone mineral density than men throughout life and experience an accelerated rate of bone loss following the menopause. By age 75 years, a woman may have lost 50% of her bone mass, while a man will have only lost 25% of bone mass by age 90 years.

Because of postmenopausal osteoporosis, the fracture rate in post-menopausal women is greater than that in age-matched men. The female to male ratio for true fracture incidence varies from site to site in the skeleton from 2 to 1 at the femoral neck to at least 10 to 1 for the vertebral crush fracture. The large number of elderly women in the population results in about 80% of all cases of hip fracture occurring in women who are mostly over age 65 years.

3.46 What is the association between osteoporosis and the menopause?

The rate of bone loss accelerates after the menopause because of the increase in bone resorption. While the relative loss of trabecular bone exceeds that of cortical bone, menopause has an adverse effect upon both spinal (predominantly trabecular) and hip (predominantly cortical) bone density. The rate of loss of spinal trabecular bone during the first 5 years after natural menopause may be as much as 5% per annum; after oophorectomy it may be 7–9% per annum. Trabecular bone is metabolically more active and is lost faster than cortical bone possibly because of its greater surface area. The rate of loss of bone begins to decrease approximately 8–10 years after the menopause for reasons that are not fully understood. It has been reported that a woman will lose 50% of her trabecular bone density and 35% of her cortical bone density during her lifetime. When the bone density falls below a critical threshold then the risk of fracture is correspondingly increased.

3.47 What other factors affect fracture risk?

One of the most important of these is the peak bone mass achieved in adult life. Thus, postmenopausally, a woman may experience a fast rate of bone loss but may not suffer fracture because of a high, adult peak bone mass. Conversely, a woman with a slow rate of postmenopausal bone loss may

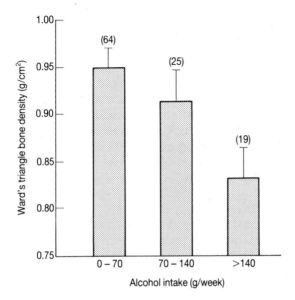

Fig. 3.4 Mean ($\pm$ SE) bone density (g/cm^2) in Ward's triangle in premenopausal women with various alcohol intakes grouped to show <1 (0–70g), 1–2 (70–140g) and >2 (>140g) standard drinks per day. Figures in brackets represent numbers in each group. (From Stevenson J C et al 1989 British Medical Journal 298: 924–928. Reproduced with permission.)

suffer fracture because her adult peak bone mass was low. While there is a correlation between peak bone mass and subsequent rate of loss postmenopausally (the greater the former the faster the rate of loss), our present understanding is that this may not be sufficiently close to predict fracture risk from biochemical assessments of the rate of bone loss during the early postmenopausal years. At present, the best predictor of bone mass at age 70 years is bone mass at age 50 years. Therefore, screening during the early postmenopausal years to detect women at high risk of osteoporotic fracture in later life must involve some assessment of bone density.

Peak bone mass is largely genetically determined, hence the importance of a family history of osteoporosis in predicting fracture risk in an individual. However, it can be affected by various lifestyle factors. Those reducing peak bone mass are prolonged periods of amenorrhoea during the reproductive era, and also heavy tobacco and alcohol consumption. More than two alcoholic drinks each day reduce hip bone density by 12% in women in their late 40s (Fig. 3.4). Other lifestyle factors may increase peak bone mass. Preliminary data suggest that high parity is beneficial. The effects of exercise on peak bone density have been studied incompletely. However, to be beneficial on bone, exercise may well have to be gravity dependent

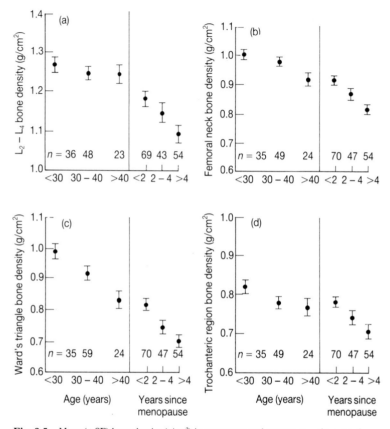

Fig. 3.5   Mean (±SE) bone density (g/cm²) in premenopausal women at various stated ages and in postmenopausal women at defined times after menopause. n = numbers of observations. (a) = L_2–L_4 vertebrae (spine); (b), (c) and (d) = various sites in the hip. (From Stevenson J C et al 1989 British Medical Journal 298: 924-928. Reproduced with permission.)

(walking, running but not yoga or swimming), and even then may only be of small benefit to the hip.

Peak bone density in the spine and hip is achieved by the end of or soon after linear skeletal growth (less than 20 years of age). Premenopausally, no significant decline in bone density has been observed in the spine and a slow linear decrease occurs in the hip. However, the latter is small as compared to the loss of bone at both these sites which occurs after menopause. The pre- and postmenopausal spinal and hip data are shown in Figure 3.5.

The other major factor affecting fracture risk is likelihood of falling. This will not be considered further here.

3.48 How does oestrogen influence bone turnover?

The precise mechanism whereby oestrogen prevents bone loss is still uncertain. It has been proposed that oestrogen lack permits excessive parathyroid hormone activity. However, the plasma levels of parathyroid hormone observed in postmenopausal women are not those usually associated with increased bone resorption. It has also been suggested that oestrogen controls bone resorption indirectly by regulating the secretion of calcitonin. Women have lower values of calcitonin than men and there is also an age-related decline in secretion. Calcitonin exerts a bone conserving effect on the skeleton by inhibiting osteoclastic activity. Thus, loss of ovarian function may accelerate the age-related decline in calcitonin secretion which results in an increase in bone resorption postmenopausally. Blacks have higher levels of calcitonin than whites, and this theory may help explain why osteoporosis is much less common in blacks than in whites. Furthermore, blacks have a higher peak bone mass than whites.

Alternatively, oestrogen may have a direct action on the skeleton since specific high affinity receptors for oestrogen have been found in human cultured osteoblasts. However, the receptor levels are low and, to date, the oestrogen receptor has not been found in osteoclasts. Postmenopausal osteoporosis, as stated previously, is due to an increase in bone resorption indicative of excessive osteoclastic activity.

3.49 What are the typical osteoporotic fractures?

1. Distal radius (wrist or Colles' fracture)
2. Crush fracture of thoracic and lumbar vertebrae
3. Femoral neck

3.50 How many women suffer wrist fracture?

In women, the incidence of wrist fracture begins to rise around age 50 years and increases approximately 10-fold during the postmenopause to reach 65 per 10 000 women by age 80 years. About 15% of women reaching age 75 years will have suffered a wrist fracture.

There is no corresponding increase in wrist fracture incidence in men.

3.51 How common are vertebral crush fractures?

This is the most common osteoporotic fracture. Surprisingly, data on the incidence vary widely and this most probably reflects the different criteria used to define vertebral fracture. Approximately 15% of women aged 75 years have clinical evidence of this fracture, and a further 10% have radiological evidence. Thus, some fractures appear to be silent clinically.

3.52 What are the effects?

Significant collapse of one vertebral body usually leads to severe pain of finite duration. In addition to repeated pain, numerous crush fractures result in loss of height and often a marked kyphosis (Dowager's Hump). Because movement of the thoracic cage becomes limited, cardio-pulmonary embarrassment may ensue leading to severely reduced exercise tolerance and disability.

3.53 How many women suffer hip fracture?

In 1985, 35 000 women in England and Wales sustained a fractured neck of femur, of whom 74% were over 75 years of age.

3.54 Is the incidence rising?

Yes. The incidence of fractured neck of femur has increased considerably during the past 30 years. This is due to an increase in the age specific rates as well as to an increase in the age of the population. Over the last 30 years the age specific incidence has doubled in men and women aged 65 years and over. Using current age and sex specific incidence rates for hip fracture in England and Wales, the probability that a woman will suffer a fractured hip before the age of 85 years is 12%; for a man it is 5%. The estimates may double by the year 2016 when there may be 117 000 new cases of hip fracture per year.

3.55 Why is this so?

The reason is uncertain. It has been proposed that cigarette smoking, excessive alcohol use and/or an increasingly sedentary lifestyle may be important.

3.56 Why should we be concerned about hip fractures?

The cost of hip fracture is substantial in terms of both morbidity and mortality.

Morbidity is great in terms of misery, disability and dependence with three out of every five women sustaining hip fracture being unable to return to an independent life. Mortality is also high with 20% of women who sustain hip fracture dying within one year.

3.57 What are the financial costs?

The financial cost of all osteoporotic fractures has been estimated at 700–800 million pounds per annum in the UK. Hospitalization for hip fracture is almost universal. Approximately 20% of orthopaedic beds in England and Wales are occupied by women following hip fracture. The average length of stay in hospital is approximately 30 days with only a minority of patients regaining their former mobility. Large numbers require long-term nursing care and/or sheltered accommodation.

Osteoporosis thus presents a formidable clinical and financial problem and a potentially devastating drain on National Health Service resources.

3.58 Are all women at risk of osteoporosis?

If all women were to live long enough then the answer would be yes. However, with the current female life expectancy the answer must be no. Screening early postmenopausal women to detect those at greatest risk for later osteoporotic fracture is considered further in Question 5.29.

3.59 What are the risk factors for osteoporosis?

These are shown in Table 3.2. It is emphasized that these factors have been derived from studies of large populations. The value of these risk factors in determining risk in the individual woman is highly questionable. For example, we have patients with every risk factor in whom bone density measurements have shown satisfactory skeletal preservation in both the spine and hip. Conversely, we have patients with no risk factor in whom significant spinal and hip bone density has been lost within 1−2 years of menopause. The table is included more for the sake of completeness rather than with a recommendation that it is clinically useful.

3.60 What is the evidence that female sex steroids influence arterial disease risk?

This comes from various sources. Epidemiological studies have reported that at around age 40−50 years many more men than women die from arterial disease (particularly myocardial infarction). The male excess rapidly diminishes thereafter and by age 75-80 years the death rates between the sexes are similar. There are two explanations for this. Firstly, that the male population possesses a sub-group at very high risk for arterial disease (perhaps, genetically determined). The majority die by age 50 years leaving only those at low risk. The second explanation is that premenopausal women are protected against arterial disease. Following menopause, this protection is lost and death rates in postmenopausal women rise and eventually reach those seen in the male population.

Table 3.2   Factors affecting risk of osteoporosis

Age
Premature menopause
Time since menopause
Racial origin
Family history
Height and weight
Gravidity
Parity
Use of oral contraceptives
Cigarette consumption
Alcohol intake
Sedentary lifestyle
Calcium intake
Use of oral steroids
Hyperthyroid disease
Caffeine intake

(From Stevenson J C et al 1989 British Medical Journal 298: 924–928.
Reproduced with permission.)

Evidence to support the second explanation has come from various epidemiological studies: some of these data are reproduced in Figure 3.6. After controlling for age (which is the most important predictor of arterial disease risk), postmenopausal women were found to be at excess risk as compared to their premenopausal counterparts. The importance of premature menopause in increasing arterial disease risk (a two-fold increase) is discussed in Question 5.9 and illustrated in Figure 5.3. Thus, loss of ovarian function appears to increase arterial disease risk.

3.61 Why is arterial disease so important in women?

Because it is the commonest cause of death in women aged over 50 years and kills approximately one woman in four (see Question 1.6 and Figures 1.3 and 1.4). Because it is so common, any major effect of HRT in reducing arterial disease risk is likely to be of considerable financial benefit.

3.62 What are the possible mechanisms whereby oestrogen lack may increase arterial disease risk?

These are poorly understood and we will classify them as 'lipid' and 'non-lipid' mechanisms.

Whilst puberty appears to have little effect on plasma lipid and lipoprotein concentrations, loss of ovarian function following premature surgical or natural menopause causes profound changes in lipid and lipoprotein metabolism. Due most probably to differences in study design,

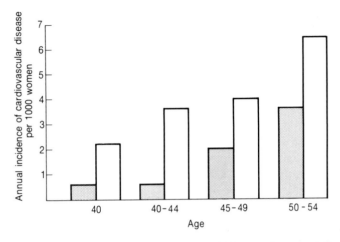

Fig. 3.6   Annual incidence of cardiovascular disease per 1000 women by menopausal status. ▨ = premenopausal; ☐ = postmenopausal. (Adapted from Gordon T, Kannel WB, Hjortland MC et al 1978 Annals of Internal Medicine 89: 157–161. Reproduced with permission.)

and cohort and laboratory differences, the data are not entirely consistent but most authorities accept that ovarian failure is followed by an increase in total cholesterol due, principally, to a rise in the low density lipoprotein (LDL)-cholesterol sub-fraction. The effects on high density lipoprotein (HDL)-cholesterol are more controversial with some studies reporting no change but others a reduction in plasma concentrations following menopause. Data on the principal HDL-cholesterol sub-fractions, HDL_2 and HDL_3, are much more sparse: preliminary data suggest that the former is reduced and that HDL_3-cholesterol levels rise after menopause. Plasma triglyceride values rise but these are also age-dependent.

Little is known about the non-lipid mechanisms. In lower mammals, oestradiol acts as a vasodilator on the aorta and major arteries and thus, it is biologically plausible that similar effects occur in women. There are reports that one condition which may be associated with fluctuating plasma oestradiol concentrations causing changes in arterial tone, menstrual migraine, can be helped with oestradiol supplementation. Flow velocity waveforms of the uterine artery change with time since menopause and are profoundly influenced by HRT (see Question 4.35), and preliminary data indicate identical changes within the internal carotid artery. The presence of a protein associated to the oestradiol receptor has been identified in the muscularis of human, premenopausal arteries, and thus it is possible that oestrogens influence arterial tone through a conventional, sex steroid-receptor mediated mechanism. However, oestrogens may also influence arterial status through non-receptor mediated mechanisms by changing prostaglandin, glycosaminoglycans and collagen metabolism: they may also influence blood pressure.

3.63 Are the lipid changes which follow loss of ovarian function likely to increase arterial disease risk?

Yes, with one important caveat. The overwhelming majority of studies correlating arterial disease risk and the lipid profile have been performed in men, and far fewer data are available for women. If the sexes respond similarly to lipid and lipoprotein concentrations, then the rises in total and LDL-cholesterol and the fall in HDL_2-cholesterol which follow loss of ovarian function will be atherogenic because such a profile (low HDL_2/LDL ratio) is associated with an increase in arterial disease risk in men. As discussed later (see Question 4.34), there is evidence that lipid and lipoprotein changes are important in women. However, the impact of a potentially atherogenic lipid and lipoprotein profile in women may be modified by the presence of oestrogen. For example, in non-human primates fed a high cholesterol diet, administration of an oral contraceptive formulation containing an oestrogen and an androgenic progestogen which lowered HDL and elevated LDL-cholesterol did not increase arterial disease as determined at necropsy.

4. The benefits of hormone replacement therapy (HRT)

During the last few years considerable evidence has accumulated that hormone replacement therapy (HRT) relieves the acute symptoms of oestrogen deficiency, beneficially affects some of the intermediate symptoms, and reduces the risk of some of the long-term sequalae. Thus, HRT can fulfil both therapeutic and preventive roles.

4.1 Which acute and intermediate symptoms respond to HRT?

Some of the controversy that surrounds HRT stems from the diversity of symptoms claimed by some to respond to HRT. It must be remembered that postmenopausal women are highly placebo responsive. Therefore, conclusions drawn from uncontrolled studies are of little value.

Placebo-controlled studies have consistently reported that oestrogens relieve vasomotor instability, insomnia and the symptoms of lower genital tract atrophy. With regard to the psychological status, the reported benefits vary widely and these discrepancies may be due to differences in trial design. However, data are available from large-scale double-blind, randomized, placebo-controlled, cross-over studies which reported beneficial psychological effects with HRT.

4.2 What are the benefits of oestrogen therapy on vasomotor symptoms?

There is evidence from the studies referred to above that oestrogens are more effective than placebo in relieving vasomotor symptoms. All types of oestrogen therapy will give relief if an adequate plasma oestrogen concentration is obtained. The latter can be readily achieved by the oral, subcutaneous and transdermal routes but is more difficult with the vaginal route of administration. See Chapter 6.

4.3 How quickly can relief of flushes be achieved?

The response to treatment can be dramatic with a marked effect obvious within a few days and elimination of flushing achieved within a few weeks.

However, the more usual response is more gradual. Most studies have shown a continuing improvement during the first three months of treatment. Therefore, it is important to continue treatment for at least this long before concluding that a certain dose of oestrogen is inadequate.

4.4 Is this just a short-term phenomenon?

No. Once stabilized on HRT, symptom relief is usually sustained throughout the treatment period. In our experience, various factors can, however, result in a partial return of vasomotor symptoms. These include a sudden increase in ambient temperature ('hot spells') during the English summer, travelling to the sun for the summer holidays, prolonged use of antibiotics which may interfere with oestrogen metabolism, and times of domestic or work stress. Abrupt cessation of therapy often results in a return of flushes and sweats. This can be avoided by a gradual reduction in oestrogen dosage over several weeks or months. See Question 10.9.

4.5 How does oestrogen compare with other treatments?

There are few comparative studies from which to draw conclusions. Oestrogen is significantly more effective than clonidine in relieving hot flushes, and has the additional benefit of improving psychological symptoms. In patients in whom oestrogens are contraindicated, progestogens may be effective. Placebo-controlled studies have shown significant benefits with oral norethisterone and with medroxyprogesterone acetate given either orally or by depo-intramuscular injection. The effects of oral norethisterone are illustrated in Figure 4.1. The mode of action of progestogens is not clear.

We are unaware of any scientifically valid studies which have reported that hypnotics, sedatives and tranquillizers are of benefit in relieving vasomotor disturbances or psychological symptoms. We believe that their use in women with typical oestrogen-deficiency complaints is difficult to justify.

4.6 How strong is the evidence for a beneficial effect of oestrogen on sleep?

There is both subjective and objective evidence that oestrogen therapy relieves sleep disturbances related to oestrogen deficiency.

Subjective data from large placebo-controlled, cross-over studies have shown significant improvements in insomnia. This is not surprising because objective measurements of finger temperature and skin resistance, and the use of continuous EEG monitoring during sleep in untreated

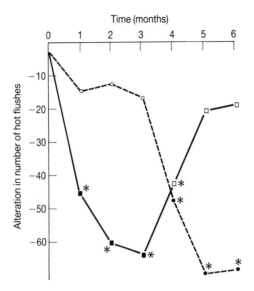

Fig. 4.1. Alteration in number of hot flushes at each month of treatment with norethisterone 5 mg/day. A randomized, double-blind, placebo-controlled study with a cross-over at 3 months (○‒‒‒● = placebo/active: ■▭▭▭▭□ = active/placebo). Asterisk indicates p < 0.01; treatment versus pre-treatment. (From Paterson M et al 1982 British Journal of Obstetrics and Gynaecology 89: 464–472. Reproduced with permission.)

postmenopausal women have shown that hot flushes at night are preceded by waking episodes, and that there is a reduction in the duration of rapid eye movement (REM) sleep. Oestrogen therapy abolishes hot flushes and the associated waking episodes; it also decreases sleep latency (the time taken to go to sleep), and increases REM sleep. Thus, the use of oestrogen therapy is more physiological than the use of sedatives or hypnotics.

4.7 Which psychological symptoms respond to oestrogen therapy?

Most placebo-controlled, double-blind studies have shown significant decreases in psychological complaints such as irritability, fatigue, anxiety and depression when oestrogen is given alone or in combination with a progestogen.

Improvements with oestrogen therapy over placebo for a variety of psychological symptoms have been reported although various authors have disagreed about the most appropriate method for assessing psychological changes. In a placebo-controlled, cross-over study of 4 months' duration which involved 64 patients with severe symptoms, oestrogen was found to be significantly more effective than placebo in alleviating not only hot flushes, insomnia and vaginal dryness but also irritability, poor memory, anxiety, worry about age, worry about self, optimism and good spirits. It was felt that the psychological improvements were secondary to the relief of disabling vasomotor symptoms, i.e. the 'domino effect' was operating. However, when an analysis was made of the 20 patients who had not reported hot flushes, certain variables (poor memory, anxiety, worry about age and self) continued to be significantly improved by oestrogens. These benefits observed in non-flushing women suggest a direct positive effect of oestrogen on the mental status.

Another large, double-blind, placebo-controlled, cross-over study investigated women who had undergone hysterectomy and bilateral oophorectomy for benign disease. This study measured the separate effects of oestrogen and progestogen and compared these with placebo. Each subject received three months of oestrogen alone, progestogen alone, oestrogen and progestogen, and placebo in random order. Oestrogen alone was found to have the most beneficial effect on the psychological status as measured by Hamilton scores, and by ordinal ratings of general wellbeing, depression, fatigue, anxiety, irritability and insomnia. Combination oestrogen/progestogen was next in beneficial effect, with progestogen alone scoring slightly better than placebo. These results are illustrated in Figure 4.2. While some of the benefits on mood were related to the relief of hot flushes, a direct psychotrophic effect of oestrogen was also suggested.

These studies concord with previous work which described a mental tonic effect of exogenous oestrogens. It has been suggested that this improved feeling of wellbeing may reflect a pharmacological effect of oestrogen, rather than reversal of a postmenopausal phenomenon. However, the plasma oestrogen levels achieved with HRT are well within the premenopausal range (see Chapter 6), and therefore we believe that a pharmacological effect is unlikely.

4.8 What are the effects of adding progestogen?

When a progestogen is added to oestrogen the beneficial effects on mood are reduced. This disadvantage of progestogens is discussed further in Question 7.8.

4.9 What are the observed benefits of oestrogen on the lower genital tract?

Placebo-controlled, cross-over studies have demonstrated that oestrogen therapy is effective in relieving vaginal dryness. Provided that the oestrogen dose is adequate, the premenopausal maturation index (which measures the

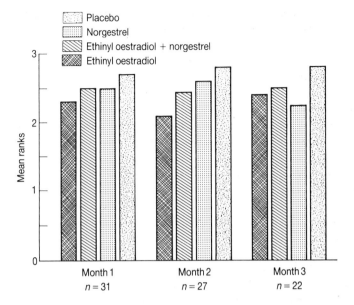

Fig. 4.2 Hormone therapy and mood. Higher ranks indicate increasing feelings of depression. n = number of patients. (From Dennerstein L et al 1979 Maturitas 2: 253–259. Reproduced with permission.)

percentage of parabasal, intermediate and superficial cells observed in a vaginal smear) can be restored.

The oestrogen dose required to treat the symptoms of lower genital tract atrophy is usually less than that required for the treatment of vasomotor symptoms. Progestogens alone are not an effective alternative for the treatment of lower genital tract atrophy.

4.10 Does oestrogen therapy improve libido and sexual functioning?

In controlled studies oestrogen replacement therapy has been shown to improve vaginal dryness, coital satisfaction and sexual desire. Data on the effects on frequency of coitus and orgasm are inconsistent. Oestrogen therapy appears to increase desire and satisfaction primarily through its pronounced effect on vaginal lubrication.

It remains difficult to distinguish the relative contributions of ageing and oestrogen deprivation to decreased libido and other markers of sexual functioning. Studies have failed to demonstrate that oophorectomy has a universally adverse effect on sexual functioning. The importance of psychological factors and the contribution made by the partner must not be overlooked.

In the absence of local vaginal problems, some studies have reported that oestrogen replacement is of little benefit in the treatment of decreased or absent libido.

4.11 What are the effects of adding testosterone?

Here the studies are inconsistent. Some workers have failed to demonstrate any difference in effect between oestrogen given by itself and oestrogen plus testosterone. Others have found that the addition of the testosterone enhances sexual desire, and have recommended the routine addition of testosterone implants for patients with loss of libido.

Because of this discrepancy, no clear guidelines can be recommended for routine clinical practice. While many patients respond well to oestrogen alone, in our experience there are definitely some whose libido will only improve when testosterone is added.

4.12 Do progestogens have less favourable effects on libido and sexual functioning?

In our experience, the addition of a progestogen to the oestrogen may reduce the beneficial effects on sexual functioning. The mechanism of action is unclear but recently published data suggest that progestogens reduce vulval blood flow. Thus, it is likely that they will oppose oestrogen benefits on vaginal lubrication. This may be the mechanism whereby certain oral contraceptive formulations cause vaginal dryness leading to reduced libido.

4.13 What are the beneficial effects of oestrogen on urinary symptoms?

Oestrogen therapy may be effective in the treatment of the urethral syndrome (frequency, urgency and dysuria in the absence of urinary tract infection). Some studies have been able to correlate symptomatic improvements with changes in urethral cytology in postmenopausal women, and have shown that both respond to oestrogen therapy. Improvements may be reported after 1–2 weeks of treatment, and after therapy is stopped women may remain asymptomatic for four weeks to six months but their symptoms usually ultimately recur. For this reason, many patients will require long-term oestrogen therapy to provide adequate relief of symptoms.

The urethral syndrome is not specifically related to the climacteric and it is unlikely that it has a single aetiology. Hormone therapy alone will correct the atrophic urethritis but may not give complete relief of voiding difficulties if these are related more to gross anatomical derangements, e.g. prolapse.

It has recently been shown that urinary symptoms are common in women presenting to a hospital menopause clinic with climacteric symptoms. Between 30 and 50% reported symptoms of stress incontinence, frequency, nocturia and urgency. This study showed no statistically significant difference between the peri- and postmenopausal women for any of these symptoms, and this suggests that either oestrogen deprivation has no effect on lower urinary tract symptomatology or that urological changes occur as an early event in the climacteric process. Subsequently, the same authors showed a statistically significant improvement in every symptom (except for urgency) after 3 months of oestrogen replacement therapy. Unfortunately, this study was not placebo-controlled.

Other controlled studies have reported that oestrogens improve urinary frequency. However, the authors commented that this improvement could be due to a direct effect of the oestrogen upon the urinary tract, or due to an indirect effect mediated through less sleep disturbance.

4.14 Can oestrogens be used to treat urinary incontinence?

Several studies have reported improvements in stress incontinence in up to 50% of postmenopausal women treated with oestrogens for several weeks. The following are known to influence urinary continence: urethral mucosa thickness, intra-abdominal location of the proximal urethra, and peri-urethral muscle tension. Continence is maintained if the maximum urethral pressure exceeds the bladder pressure.

Oestrogens have been shown to increase the number of superficial cells in the urethral epithelium, i.e. a more mature picture results. Oestrogens have also been shown to increase blood flow through the vascular plexuses underlying the urethral epithelium. Urodynamic studies have shown that in women with stress incontinence, the abdominal pressure transmission to the proximal urethra at the time of stress improves significantly following vaginal oestrogen therapy. This may be due to an overall increase in collagen content of the connective tissue surrounding the urethra and bladder neck. In addition, oestrogen therapy may enhance contractions of the striated peri-urethral muscle fibres at the time of stress. One study has reported that oestrogens potentiate the effect of alpha-adrenergic drugs on the urethra in postmenopausal women.

4.15 What are the effects of oestrogen therapy on the skin?

Many postmenopausal women complain of generalized dry, flaky skin, brittle nails and dry hair. These symptoms tend to improve with HRT

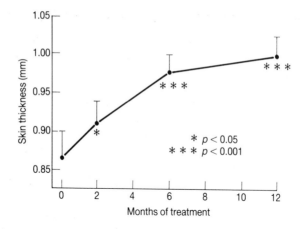

Fig. 4.3 Mean ($\pm$ SE) skin thickness during 12 months' therapy with oestradiol and testosterone implants, 100 mg, reinserted every 6 months. (From Brincat M et al 1985 British Journal of Obstetrics and Gynaecology 92: 256–259. Reproduced with permission.)

although therapy has to be given for some months. Until recently many of these changes were thought to be part of the ageing process but it is becoming apparent that sex hormones affect the skin. (See Question 3.37 and Fig. 3.3)

Both oestrogen and androgen receptors have been identified on fibroblasts in the skin. Oestrogens have been shown to influence fibroblast function by increasing the rate of collagen production, and the hydroscopic qualities of collagen fibres in connective tissues. This leads to an increase in dermal water content. Skin thickness and skin collagen content decline after the menopause but can be restored to normal premenopausal levels with oestrogen or oestrogen and testosterone replacement therapy. These changes are shown in Figure 4.3. It appears that skin thickness and skin collagen content are related to the number of years after menopause rather than the chronological age.

While many women report improvements in skin and hair texture with HRT there is no evidence that such treatment retards the development of skin wrinkles. However, the benefits of oestrogens upon the skin with respect to general skin health and in particular healing (for example after surgery) have not been studied.

Some climacteric women report a sensation of crawling feelings over the skin (formication). We have observed that this symptom can respond to oestrogen therapy (see Question 3.37).

4.16 What other symptoms may be related to collagen content?

Some women report joint pains and myalgia for the first time around the menopause. In our experience, the joints that typically become troublesome are the metacarpal, wrist, elbow and shoulders. The weight-bearing joints seem to be affected less commonly. Again, in our experience, HRT may be beneficial and there are preliminary data reporting that the incidence of various types of arthritis is significantly reduced in postmenopausal oestrogen users as compared to non-users. This effect may reflect an oestrogen associated improvement in collagen content of ligaments and other connective tissues. Similarly, some women find that backache is improved with at least 6 months' treatment with HRT, and one placebo-controlled study has confirmed this.

We have seen women who have reported shrinkage and bleeding from the gums which starts during the climacteric. In our limited experience, these symptoms sometimes resolve with HRT. However, the association between the oestrogen status and peridontal resorption is controversial. We have other patients who have developed a dry mouth and dry eyes during the climacteric; the response to oestrogen therapy has been variable.

The relationship between oestrogens and loss of hair is poorly understood. This may be age-dependent rather than a hormone-dependent problem.

OSTEOPOROSIS

4.17 How should oestrogens be used in osteoporosis?

At present, oestrogens have an established role in the prevention of osteoporosis. They may also be beneficial in treating established disease.

It is well recognized that the treatment of established disease is difficult because of the lack of a non-toxic agent which will stimulate new bone formation. The primary problem with established disease is that (based upon our current understanding) trabeculae that have been destroyed cannot be reinstated. At the microanatomic level, increased postmenopausal bone resorption leads initially to erosion and eventually to loss of the trabecular plates which are integral to bone strength. These changes are shown in Figure 4.4. Because of the relationship between bone mass and fracture rate (see Fig. 5.5), any therapy which may increase bone density moderately in the remaining trabeculae in women with established disease may reduce later fracture risk in that individual. Thus, preventing further bone loss may have a beneficial effect even in women with established disease.

Various anti-resorptive agents can prevent postmenopausal loss of bone.

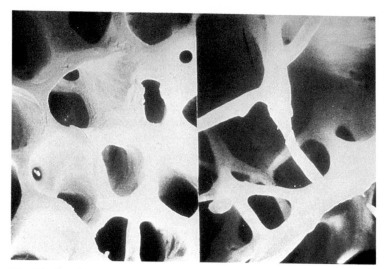

Fig. 4.4   Scanning electron micrograph of trabecular bone showing normal bone on left and osteoporotic bone on right. (Dempster D W et al 1986 Journal of Bone Mineral Research 1: 15–21. Reproduced with permission.)

These include the calcitonins and the bisphosphonates. The former have the disadvantage of having to be administered by injection until intranasal delivery systems become more widely available. Only preliminary data are available on the bisphosphonates but they are encouraging.

4.18 What is the evidence for the use of oestrogen to prevent osteoporosis?

Regrettably, there are few data upon the effects of HRT in women with established disease. The scant results that are available show that oestrogens can improve bone density slightly, and appear to reduce fracture risk. Thus, importantly, even patients with established disease may benefit from HRT.

There is widespread agreement from numerous prospective, placebo-controlled studies that oestrogens prevent bone loss in early postmenopausal women, both post-oophorectomy and after natural menopause. Longitudinal studies have demonstrated significant protection at the metacarpal, radius and vertebrae using a variety of measurement techniques. Because the technique for measuring bone density at the hip accurately has only recently been introduced, only sparse longitudinal data are available for this site. However, data from one group have shown that bone mineral density of the femoral neck (as measured by dual photon absorptiometry) is significantly greater in the group treated with oestrogen than in untreated women (see Fig 4.7).

Many studies have reported that long-term oestrogen therapy reduces the risk of fracture at the hip, wrist and spine.

Oestrogens have a major role to play in the prevention of postmenopausal osteoporosis. It is clear that oestrogens conserve bone mass at all skeletal sites and can reduce the incidence of osteoporotic fracture.

4.19 How do oestrogens conserve bone density?

Oestrogens decrease the rate of bone resorption, principally by an inhibition of osteoclastic activity. This property is shared with other anti-resorptive agents such as the calcitonins. There is some evidence that oestrogens also correct the imbalance between resorption and bone formation at each bone remodelling site. Thus, oestrogens reverse the changes seen after the loss of ovarian function by restoring the number of remodelling sites to pre-menopausal levels, and correcting the imbalance between resorption and formation at each remodelling site.

Small increases in bone mass are often seen when oestrogen therapy is initiated. These increments are small and subsequently level off. In the early stages of oestrogen treatment bone resorption is inhibited and there is a decrease in the activation of new bone remodelling sites. However, bone formation continues at previously existing remodelling sites and thus, bone mass increases slightly until a new steady state is achieved.

Using biochemical markers of bone turnover oestrogens have been shown to reverse the changes which occur at the menopause. Following administration of oestrogens both plasma total and ionized calcium and phosphate fall together with fasting urinary calcium/creatinine and hydroxyproline/creatinine ratios (biochemical markers of bone turnover). Similarly, there are decreases in serum alkaline phosphatase and serum bone Gla protein (osteocalcin). Finally, there is a rise in the calculated renal tubular maximal reabsorption of calcium and a fall in that of phosphate.

Some of the mechanisms whereby oestrogens may exert their effects on bone have been referred to in Chapter 3. There is considerable evidence that oestrogens act indirectly by stimulating calcitonin secretion. They may also oppose the bone resorbing actions of parathyroid hormone and 1,25-dihydroxy vitamin D. Oestrogens may also influence the proliferation of osteoblasts, possibly via the production of growth factors such as insulin-like growth factor 1 (IGF-1) (formerly somatomedin), and transforming growth factor beta (TGF-beta). The effects of oestrogens on TGF-beta and on prostaglandins may lead to inhibition of bone resorption by suppressing the differentiation of osteoclasts from their bone marrow pre-cursors. Finally, oestrogens may exert a direct effect on bone cells via bone oestrogen receptors.

4.20 Does HRT reduce fracture rates?

Epidemiological studies have shown that HRT protects against fractures of the wrist, spine and hip. Six retrospective case-controlled studies have reported reductions in fracture rates of the wrist and hip of between 50−60% with postmenopausal use of oestrogens. In general, greater benefits have been observed in those oestrogen-treated women who began therapy soon after menopause and had received treatment for more than 5 years.

A retrospective cohort study reported a 50% reduction in the prevalence of vertebral and wrist fractures in oestrogen-takers compared with never-users. Similarly, a retrospective cohort study of nearly 3000 women in the North East corner of the USA reported a relative risk of hip fracture in ever-users of 0.65 after adjustment for age and weight. For women who had taken oestrogens within the previous 2 years this relative risk was further reduced to 0.34. Taking oestrogens within 4 years of menopause protected against fracture, and recent use of oestrogens appeared to be as protective in women under age 65 years as compared to those aged 65−74 years. This is one of the few studies to investigate fracture frequency in older HRT users.

Data on vertebral compression fractures are more sparse. However, one prospective, double-blind, placebo-controlled trial which extended for 10 years reported that the placebo-treated group had a higher incidence of vertebral compression fractures and had experienced a significant reduction in height as compared to the oestrogen-treated women.

The observed reductions in risk are in good agreement with those calculated from mathematical models. For example, it has been calculated that 5 years of use of HRT will give a 50% reduction in hip fracture incidence. This is illustrated in Figure 4.5. Other groups have calculated that 10 years of adequate HRT administered soon after menopause to the 25% of the population with lowest bone mass at this time will achieve a 45% reduction in femoral neck fracture.

4.21 When should treatment with hormone replacement therapy start?

To maximize the potential benefits of HRT on the skeleton, treatment should be started in the late perimenopausal or early postmenopausal years. Therapy must be targeted towards prevention of the accelerated phase of bone loss which occurs during the first few years after natural or surgical menopause. The effects of starting oestrogens at different times following surgical menopause are illustrated in Figure 4.6, Clearly, maximum benefits

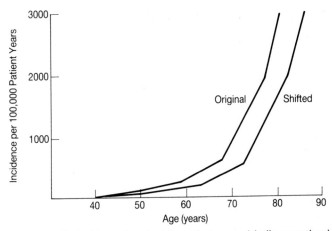

Fig. 4.5 Age-specific incidence of proximal femur fracture as originally reported and as it might appear if osteoporosis onset were delayed or progression slowed sufficiently to shift the rate to an age group five years older. (Adapted from Melton J 1988 In: Zichella L, Whitehead M I, van Keep P A (eds) The climacteric and beyond. Parthenon, Carnforth pp 127-129. Reproduced with permission).

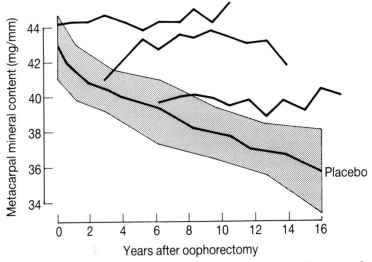

Fig. 4.6 Effect on metacarpal bone mineral density of starting oestrogen at different times after oophorectomy as compared with placebo (shaded). (From Lindsay R, Hart DM, Abdalla H, Al Azzawi F, 1987 In: Christiansen C, Johansen JS, Riis BJ (eds) Osteoporosis 1987. Osteopress, Copenhagen pp. 508–512. Reproduced with permission.)

were observed when oestrogens were started immediately after or within 3 years of oophorectomy. Under these circumstances, bone mass was completely maintained. However, starting treatment 6 years after oophorectomy still conserved bone mass at the pre-treatment level, although the bone loss that had occurred between 3 and 6 years after oophorectomy was not reversed. Thus, bone loss may be arrested by oestrogens started at any stage after loss of ovarian function. While the benefits to the patient in terms of reduced fracture risk may be greatest in those women commencing oestrogen treatment within the first few years after menopause, starting oestrogens many years after menopause may reduce later risk of fracture. We can only re-state that more data upon the effects on fracture risk of starting oestrogens many years after menopause are urgently required.

4.22 How long should HRT be continued?

There is general agreement that HRT should be continued for at least 5 years after the menopause to gain a 50% reduction in hip fracture risk and perhaps a slightly greater reduction in vertebral fracture risk. This assumes an age at menopause of approximately 50 years. Women undergoing a premature menopause would need to take HRT for longer periods of time, starting soon after menopause and continuing up to age 55 years.

It is not known whether extending the duration of HRT administration, for example up to 10 years, will exert greater protective effects.

4.23 What is the effect of stopping oestrogen therapy?

While there seems little doubt that bone loss is prevented or dramatically reduced during oestrogen administration, the effect is reversible. Bone loss resumes after oestrogen withdrawal.

The precise rate of bone loss after stopping oestrogen treatment remains uncertain. One study reported an accelerated loss of bone following oestrogen withdrawal and thereby concluded that short-term therapy of between two and four years had no lasting beneficial effect on bone mass. However, this study was performed exclusively on castrates. Another study, which investigated only women who had undergone natural menopause, reported that bone loss following withdrawal of oestrogen therapy was not accelerated, but was similar to the rate of bone loss occurring in untreated women. Thus, the observed differences between the studies may simply reflect the different populations of women who were investigated. Bone loss appears to be accelerated after castration as compared to that occurring after natural menopause.

4.24 For how long do oestrogens reduce fracture risk after treatment is withdrawn?

Few clinical data are available to answer this question. Predictions from models are discussed in Question 4.20 and illustrated in Figure 4.5.

4.25 What dose of oestrogen is required to prevent osteoporosis?

It is often stated that the minimum requirement is 0.625 mg of conjugated equine oestrogens orally per day or 2 mg of oestradiol orally, daily. A 50 mg oestradiol implant is also effective. However, two caveats must be added. Firstly, the majority of dose-ranging studies have been performed upon the peripheral skeleton (metacarpal and wrist), and it is not clear whether it is valid to extrapolate responses of the peripheral skeleton to the central skeleton (spine and hip). Secondly, the few dose-ranging studies that have measured spinal bone density have reported that bone conservation is not achieved in a minority of women with these doses. For example, conjugated equine oestrogens 0.625 mg daily was not an effective spinal bone conserver in approximately 30% of women after oophorectomy and in approximately 25% of women after natural menopause. The reasons for this lack of effect are not clear. It could be due to a failure of compliance or it may mean that some women require higher doses for skeletal preservation.

Similar unpublished data are available for the hip. Effective bone conservation was not achieved in approximately 15% of women taking this dose of this oral preparation.

Transdermal administration of oestradiol from 'patches' is a relatively recent introduction and, therefore, there are few long-term studies reporting the effects of this route on the postmenopausal skeleton. Recently-published studies have shown that transdermal oestradiol 50 μg daily has identical effects to conjugated equine oestrogens 0.625 mg daily (Fig. 4.7). Effective bone conservation has been observed in the spine in approximately 95% of women taking these preparations: the transdermal system failed to conserve hip bone density effectively in approximately 15% of women.

Further research is needed to establish why some women fail to respond to oral and transdermal oestrogens.

4.26 What are the effects of progestogens on the skeleton?

There was concern that the addition of a progestogen to the oestrogen therapy might oppose the beneficial effects of the latter on bone mass. This fear is without substantiation and properly conducted, placebo-controlled trials have shown that combined oestrogen/progestogen regimens conserve bone mass.

There is some evidence that progestogens, given by themselves, can exert a protective effect on the skeleton. Short-term studies using either bone density measurements or biochemical markers of bone turnover have shown that certain progestogens can prevent bone loss. Some workers have suggested that progestogens increase bone formation but this has not been confirmed. Progestogens are believed to compete for glucocorticoid receptors

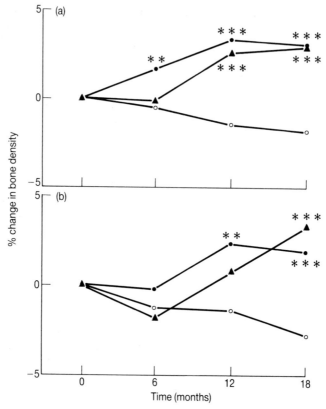

Fig. 4.7 Effects of oral therapy (conjugated equine oestrogens 0.625 mg/day and levonorgestrel 150 μg for 12 days each 28-day cycle (Prempak-C®: Wyeth-Ayerst) and transdermal hormone replacement therapy [oestradiol 50 μg/day (Estraderm®: Ciba-Geigy) for 14 days followed by a combined patch delivering oestradiol 50 μg/day and norethisterone acetate approximately 250 μg/day for 14 days] on spinal (a) and hip bone density (b), as compared to untreated women over 18 months. ● = transdermal, ▲ = oral, ○ = untreated ** P < 0.01; *** P < 0.001 versus untreated women. (From Stevenson JC et al 1990 Lancet 335: 265–269. Reproduced with permission.)

in bone, and glucocorticoids may act directly or indirectly on osteoblasts.

As yet, it is unclear whether this property of bone conservation is shared by all progestogens. For example, there is one report that norgestrel is not effective. At present, there are no data on the long-term effects of progestogen-only treatment on bone mass, nor on fracture frequency.

Nevertheless, for women who cannot or do not want to take oestrogen therapy there may be some benefits in terms of bone protection from progestogens prescribed alone. In our experience, the patient who may benefit most from progestogen-only therapy is the woman with concerns about osteoporosis in whom oestrogens are an absolute contraindication and in whom vasomotor symptoms are troublesome. In this situation, progestogens may exert dual benefits (conservation of bone and relief of flushes and sweats).

At present, there is no evidence that the addition of progestogens enhances the skeletal response to oestrogens when bone protective doses of the latter are used. However, the possibility that certain (or all) progestogens enhance the effects of oestrogen, possibly by stimulating bone formation, cannot be excluded and the results of further research are awaited.

4.27 How does HRT compare with other agents?

Various other therapeutic agents have been claimed to prevent osteoporosis and its related fractures. However, prospective, randomized studies have clearly demonstrated that oestrogens are more effective than calcium supplementation, sodium fluoride, vitamin D, 1 α vitamin D and thiazide diuretics. These data are illustrated in Figure 4.8.

There is some evidence that calcitonin therapy may be as effective as oestrogen in preventing postmenopausal bone loss. Combining the two treatments does not result in enhanced skeletal effects. Long-term studies of calcitonin have not been completed and there are no data showing a decrease in fracture rates. However, it may well be that calcitonin therapy is an acceptable alternative to oestrogen for some women, although its use may be limited to those lacking other menopausal symptoms.

The bisphosphonates are currently under investigation for the treatment of osteoporosis and preliminary results are encouraging.

4.28 Can calcium supplementation prevent osteoporosis?

This is an immensely controversial topic. The evidence that calcium supplements are an effective means of preventing the accelerated phase of bone loss occurring immediately following the menopause is conflicting. Some studies have reported benefits with calcium supplements although there is agreement that these are not as great as those seen with oestrogen therapy. However, other studies have failed to demonstrate any beneficial calcium effect at the clinically relevant sites. Thus, calcium supplementation should not be considered as an alternative to oestrogen therapy in preventing early postmenopausal bone loss.

Evidence that a minimum daily calcium intake is required for skeletal protection has come from studies of calcium balance. The most widely quoted investigation was performed in a group of nuns and reported that approximately 1500 mg of calcium was required daily in postmenopausal

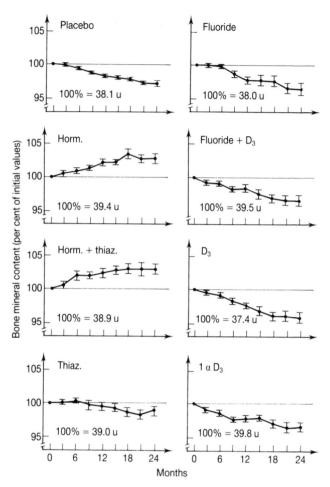

Fig. 4.8 Effects of various agents on bone mineral content in postmenopausal women. (Horm. = oestrogen/progestogen; Thiaz. = thiazide diuretics; D_3 = vitamin D; $1\alpha D_3$ = 1αvitamin D.) [Adapted from Christiansen C 1986 In: Greenblatt R (ed) A modern approach to perimenopausal years. de Gruyther, Berlin pp. 207–212. Reproduced with permission.]

women. However, it is not clear whether these data can be applied to other women with a different lifestyle. Provided that the oestrogen dose is adequate, effective spinal conservation has been reported with daily calcium intakes as low as 450 mg.

One study has suggested that the minimum dose of oestrogen required for bone conservation can be reduced when calcium is added as a supplement. Unfortunately, this study did not include an appropriate control group and confirmation of this observation is still awaited.

4.29 Does calcium intake influence peak bone mass?

Dietary calcium intake may be a factor in the attainment of peak bone mass. Therefore, children and adolescents should be encouraged to take a diet with an adequate amount of calcium.

4.30 Is calcium beneficial in women many years postmenopausal?

There is some evidence that calcium supplements may decrease the rate of bone loss in elderly women (in the seventh and eighth decades), and it will reduce the fracture risk.

Dietary calcium deficiency is rare. Women should be advised to have an adequate dietary intake of calcium. What constitutes an adequate intake is still uncertain. However, it should be remembered that the body is capable of adapting to low and high dietary calcium intakes by normal homoeostatic mechanisms.

4.31 What is the role of exercise in preventing osteoporotic fractures?

Exercise could reduce the fracture rate through two mechanisms, by increasing bone density and/or by influencing the severity and the risk of fall.

As indicated previously (Question 3.47), the effects of exercise on peak bone density have been studied incompletely. Identical comments apply to the postmenopausal era. Preliminary data suggest that gravity dependent exercise may benefit the postmenopausal skeleton slightly. However, our current understanding is that exercise, by itself, is not as effective as oestrogens at preventing postmenopausal bone loss. Thus, exercise cannot currently be recommended as an alternative to HRT with respect to skeletal preservation.

There are a number of factors other than bone density which appear to influence fracture risk. These include the severity and frequency of falling. By improving muscle bulk and tone around the hip, exercise may reduce the severity of the fall and thereby lower the fracture risk. By improving neuromuscular coordination, exercise may reduce the risk of falling. These protective effects are largely speculative at present.

4.32 Does HRT influence arterial disease risk?

Numerous studies have investigated the relationship between HRT and arterial disease risk. The majority have come from the USA and relate principally to the use of conjugated equine oestrogens administered without a progestogen. Although extensive reviews of this literature are available, they are not widely quoted in the British medical press and, therefore, certain summary tables from an extensive and recently published review are reproduced here (Tables 4.1–4.3).

Some of the studies have been retrospective, others prospective. Some have used hospital-based control whereas others have employed community/population-based controls. The end-points have varied, with some studies investigating fatal or non-fatal heart disease, whereas a few have utilized cerebrovascular accident (CVA). Some have studied apparently healthy postmenopausal women, yet others have investigated women with coronary artery occlusion confirmed by angiography. Some of the prospective studies have included 'internal' controls whereas others have used population registry data for comparisons. However, lack of space prohibits a comprehensive review. The data from studies using hospital-based controls have been omitted because of concerns that various forms of bias may have been introduced with this type of 'control' group. These are fully discussed in the excellent review (Stampfer M J & Colditz G A, 1991 Estrogen replacement therapy and coronary heart disease: a quantitative assessment of the epidemiologic evidences. Preventive Medicine 20: 47–63) to which the interested reader is referred. To assist in the interpretation of the results from these epidemiological studies, a relative risk of below 1.0 implies protection with HRT against arterial disease risk. A relative risk of 0.6 would imply a 40% reduction in incidence, and a relative risk of 0.3 a 70% reduction, etc.

Population-based case-control studies (Table 4.1)

The eight studies which utilized this design are summarized in Table 4.1. The superscript numbers adjacent to the author refer to the citation in the review of Stampfer & Colditz. The relative risks of coronary heart disease associated with HRT from these population-based case-control studies ranged from 0.3 to 0.9. However, only Ross et al reported a reduction in risk which achieved statistical significance. Thompson et al, reporting from the UK, used a combined end-point of myocardial infarction (MI) and CVA in not only oestrogen but also oestrogen/progestogen users. The results from this study were not presented separately for MI and CVA.

Cross-sectional studies (Table 4.2)

The three studies in Table 4.2 assessed the degree of coronary artery occlusion using arteriography. Sullivan et al excluded women with mild or moderate stenosis and included only those with more than 70% occlusion.

Table 4.1 Community/population-based case-control studies of oestrogen use on risk of heart disease

Study	Age of patients (years)	Number of patients	End-point	Exposure to oestrogen	Percentage oestrogen users	Relative risk (95% CI)	
						Age-adjusted	Risk factor-adjusted
Talbott[11]	39–64 mean, 566	64 (unknown number post-menopausal)	Sudden death	Current use	5%	0.34 (0.09–1.30)†	
Pfeffer[12]	50–98 mean, 75	171	1st MI	Ever use / Current use	30% / 8.7%		0.86 (0.54–1.37) / 0.68 (0.32–1.42)
Ross[13]	Under 80 mean, 73	133	Fatal CHD	Ever use	Not given	Living control 0.43 (0.24–0.75) / Dead controls 0.57 (0.33–0.99)	No change / No change
Bain[14]	30–55	120	1st MI	Ever use / Current use	53% / 27%	0.9 (0.6–1.2) / 0.7 (0.5–1.1)	0.8 (0.6–1.3) / 0.7 (0.4–1.1)
Adam[15]	50–59	76	Fatal MI	Ever use / Current use	12% / 3%	0.65 (0.29–1.45)† / 0.97 (0.41–2.28)	
Beard[16]	40–59	86	MI or sudden death	Ever use	27%		0.55 (0.24–1.30)
Thompson[17]	45–69	603	MI and stroke	Ever use 94% past use	Oestrogen alone / Oestrogen and progesterone	1.12 (0.79–1.57) / 0.86 (0.43–1.74)	1.09 (0.65–1.82) / 1.16 (0.43–3.12)

Superscript reference numerals refer to the original publication. MI, myocardial infarction; CHD, coronary heart disease. † These figures represent the crude relative risk. (Reproduced with permission from Stampfer M J, Colditz G A 1991 Preventive Medicine 20: 47–63.)

Table 4.2 Results of cross-sectional surveys of coronary artery occlusion in women with and without postmenopausal oestrogen who had coronary angiography

Study	Age of patients (years)	Number of patients	Percentage oestrogen users/type of use	Relative risk (95% CI)	
				Age adjusted	Risk factor-adjusted
Sullivan[18]	Mean, 62.8	2188	4.4%/current	0.44 (0.29–0.67) for occlusion 70+% versus no stenosis	0.58 (0.35–0.97)
Gruchow[19]	Range, 50–75	933	15.5%/current	0.59 (0.48–0.73) moderate versus low occlusion score 0.37 (0.29–0.46) severe versus low occlusion score	
McFarland[20]	Range, 35–59	283	41%/ever	0.5 (0.3–0.8) for occlusion 70+% versus no stenosis	0.50 (no CI given)

Superscript numerals refer to the original publication. (Reproduced with permission from Stampfer M J, Colditz G A 1991 Preventive Medicine 20: 47–63.)

The age-adjusted relative risk was 0.44, and this was not greatly influenced by age. Some protection was observed in high risk groups; for example, the protective effect of HRT was stronger in those with higher as compared with lower levels of cholesterol.

Gruchow et al included a substantial minority with previous MI, approximately 32% among oestrogen users and approximately 40% among non-users. An occlusion score was derived and women were classified as having a low, moderate or severe score. The relative risk for severe coronary occlusion for current oestrogen users was 0.37, and for moderate occlusion was 0.59.

McFarland et al used an identical design to Sullivan et al, and reported similar results in women with more than 70% coronary artery occlusion.

Prospective studies (Table 4.3)

Only those with 'internal' controls (i.e. follow-up of women some of whom were taking oestrogens and some of whom were not) are summarized here (Table 4.3). Because of potential bias, the prospective studies with 'external' controls (i.e. follow-up only of women taking oestrogens whose results are then compared with national statistics) have been excluded.

Two prospective studies are worthy of special mention. The Nurses' Health Study (Stampfer et al) is the largest, prospective, cohort study to investigate the relationships between arterial disease risk and HRT. In 1976, 121 700 female registered nurses completed a questionnaire and were enrolled. A further questionnaire was completed in 1978 and 32 317 postmenopausal women without prior coronary artery disease were followed for an average of 3 years. Current users of oestrogens had a relative risk of 0.3; among past users this was 0.7. Importantly, controlling for risk factors such as hypercholesterolaemia, a family history of heart disease, hypertension, diabetes mellitus, obesity and tobacco use did not materially alter the relative risk, and there was no evidence that women at lower baseline risk were selectively being prescribed HRT.

Unlike all the other cohort studies, the Framingham Heart Study (Wilson et al) initially reported an increase in risk of cardiovascular disease among ever users of oestrogens. However, a second analysis of the Framingham data (Eaker et al) reported a non-significant protective effect of HRT among women aged 50–59 years with a relative risk of 0.38. The Framingham data are thus contradictory, and they appear to be extremely sensitive as to which assessments during the course of this study of many years' duration are used for analyses. An additional problem with the Framingham data is that in both analyses the results were adjusted for HDL-cholesterol. Generally, this is considered inappropriate because oestrogens appear to protect against

Table 4.3 Prospective studies with internal controls

Study	Age at baseline (mean or range)	Number in population	Percentage oestrogen users	Follow-up (years) (mean or range)	End-point (Number of cases)	Relative risk (95% CI)	
						Age-adjusted	Risk factor-adjusted
Potocki[21]	60–70	158	52%	10 ?	MI (4)	0.31 (0.04–2.57)†	
Hammond[24]	46.3	619	49%	1.3	CHD (58)	0.33 (0.19–0.56)†	
Nachtigall[25]	55	168	50%	10	MI (4)	0.33 (0.04–2.82)†	
Lafferty[26]	45–60 (53.7)	124	49%	3–16 (8.6)	MI (7)	0.17 (0.03–1.06)†	
Stampfer[28]	30–55	32 317	Past 18% Current 35% Ever 57%	3.3	Nonfatal MI & CHD death (90)	Past 0.7 (0.4–1.2) Current 0.3 (0.2–0.6) Ever 0.5 (0.3–0.8)	0.59 (0.33–1.06) 0.30 (0.14–0.64) 0.52 (0.34–0.80)

Table 4.3 Prospective Studies (cont)

Framingham Heart Study:

Study	Age	HRT use	Follow-up	Number	Endpoint	Result	Result
Wilson	50–84	Past 14% Current 10%	8	1234	All CVD (194) CVD death (48) MI (51)	1.76 (P<0.01)†† 1.94 (P<0.05)†† 1.87 (P<0.05)††	
Eaker	50–59 60–69	15% 8%	10	695 602	CHD, no angina (35) (51)	0.26 (0.06–1.22)††,††† 1.68 (0.71–4.00)††,†††	0.4 (P > 0.05)†† 2.2 (P > 0.05)††
Bush[39, 37]	40–69	26%	8.5	2270	CVD death (50)	0.34 (0.12–0.81)	0.37 (0.16–0.88)
Petitti[31]	18–54	Ever 44%	10–13	6093	CVD death	0.9 (0.2–3.3)	0.6 (0.3–1.1)
Criqui[32]	50–79	39%	12	1868	CHD death (87)	0.75 (0.45–1.24)	0.99 (0.59–1.67)
Henderson[33]	40–101 (median, 73)	Past 43% Current 14%	4.6	8807	MI deaths (149)	Past 0.62 (0.43–0.90) Current 0.47 (0.20–2.00) Ever 0.59 (0.42–0.82)	No change No change No change
Croft[34]	20–60	Ever 6.5%	19	Nested	MI (9)	0.8	0.8 (0.3–1.8)

Superscript reference numerals refer to the original publication. MI, myocardial infarction; CHD, coronary heart disease; CVD, cardiovascular disease. †The crude odds ratio and confidence intervals (CI) are derived from data given in the paper. ††This includes high-density lipoproteins in the regression analysis. †††These results are taken as the average of findings using examination 11 and examination 12 as baseline. (Reproduced with permission from Stampfer M J, Colditz G A 1991 Preventive Medicine 20: 47–63.)

arterial disease risk, at least in part, through beneficially influencing lipid and lipoprotein concentrations (see Questions 3.62 and 4.34).

4.33 What are the limitations of these studies?

The overwhelming majority of the studies listed in Tables 4.1–4.3 examine the effects of conjugated equine oestrogens given cyclically (without a progestogen). Too few data are available on other types of oral oestrogens and on different routes of administration for meaningful conclusions about their effects on arterial disease risk to be drawn. Furthermore, the effects of added progestogen are not known (see Question 4.36).

Whilst the majority of the epidemiological evidence reports that use of HRT reduces arterial disease risk, not all experts accept this body of evidence. Some antagonists argue that all the studies are flawed, to a greater or lesser extent, by selection bias whereby patients at high risk for arterial disease (hypercholesterolaemia, hypertension, obesity, diabetes etc) have not been prescribed oestrogens. The observed reductions in relative risk in oestrogen users are more likely due, they argue, to the low background risk rather than to the effects of therapy. However, at least three large scale studies have addressed this issue and all report that oestrogens are similarly beneficial whether prescribed to low- or high-risk women. Thus, the protagonists argue that this criticism is unfounded and it is already proven that oestrogens reduce arterial disease risk.

The only way of resolving this controversy is to mount a prospective, randomized, controlled trial. Whether this will be possible is uncertain given the logistical and financial implications. Clearly, each doctor will have to draw his or her own conclusions from the available evidence. Our opinion is that oestrogens will reduce arterial disease risk. It makes biological sense that if early loss of ovarian function increases arterial disease risk, then replacement of oestrogens will reduce it.

In Question 3.62 we discussed possible mechanisms whereby loss of ovarian function might increase arterial disease risk, and we referred to them as 'lipid' and 'non-lipid' mediators.

Loss of ovarian function (i.e. loss of endogenous oestradiol) results in changes in plasma lipid and lipoprotein concentrations which are potentially atherogenic. Provided that an adequate plasma oestradiol level is achieved, it seems reasonable to predict that HRT will reverse these lipid and lipoprotein changes.

We believe that this applies both to oral and to non-oral routes of oestrogen administration. The latter, like the ovary, deliver oestradiol into the systemic circulation. Indeed, there is a substantial, predominantly European, literature that relatively high doses of oestradiol administered non-orally by intra-muscular injection, subcutaneous implantation or as a percutaneous cream significantly reduce total and LDL-cholesterol and some studies have reported an elevation of HDL-cholesterol. Because of its relatively recent introduction, data on transdermal oestradiol are more sparse but the middle and highest dose patches, delivering 50 μg or 100 μg/day, respectively, reduce total and LDL-cholesterol, and one study of the 100 μg system has reported an elevation in HDL-cholesterol. Because the entire circulating plasma volume is cleared through the liver approximately every 5 minutes, all routes of oestrogen administration, including the non-oral, will result in hepatic effects.

Because of the 'first-pass' effect of orally administered oestrogens on hepatic metabolism (see Questions 6.4 and 6.6) it has been suggested that the oral route will result in greater lipid and lipoprotein changes than a comparable oestrogen dose administered non-orally. At present, too few data from prospective, randomized studies comparing equipotent doses of oral and non-oral oestrogens are available for this suggestion to be confirmed or refuted with confidence. Both routes suppress total and LDL-cholesterol, but the oral route may well cause slightly greater beneficial effects on HDL-cholesterol. However, the non-oral and oral routes differ in one respect: the former reduces or does not change plasma triglyceride levels. Orally administered oestrogens elevate plasma triglyceride and this effect is believed due to a pharmacological action of the oestrogen on the hepatic secretion of very-low-density lipoprotein (VLDL). Elevated triglyceride levels in men appear to be an independent risk factor for ischaemic heart disease, but it is not known whether they act similarly in women. On an empiric basis, it would seem prudent to avoid orally administered oestrogens in women with hypertriglyceridaemia. At present, it would appear that less than 50% of the protection afforded by HRT in reducing arterial disease risk is mediated through potentially favourable changes in lipid and lipoprotein metabolism.

4.34 What about 'non-lipid' mechanisms?

There is a substantial literature that oestradiol acts as a vasodilator in the aorta and major arteries of other mammalian species. The causative mechanism is unknown but possible mediators were discussed in Question 3.62. Within the last 12–18 months, considerable evidence has emerged that, in major human arteries, oestradiol influences the blood flow characteristics. This is assessed using colour flow mapping and Doppler ultrasound, and typical flow velocity waveforms obtained from the uterine artery of an untreated postmenopausal woman are shown in the Frontispiece. Administration of non-oral oestradiol for 12 days caused profound changes in the flow velocity waveform (Frontispiece). Preliminary data indicate that HRT has to be administered for a longer period to affect other arteries, but 6–9 weeks of transdermal therapy can produce identical changes within the internal carotid artery. Thus, the effects of HRT on the flow velocity waveform appear to be a generalized phenomenon and are not restricted to the pelvic vasculature.

Various measurements of the flow velocity waveform can be made. Most groups have expressed their results in terms of a pulsatility index (PI), which is believed to assess impedance to blood flow distal to the point of sampling. In both the uterine and internal carotid arteries the PI is correlated more with time since menopause than with chronological age. The longer the postmenopausal interval, the higher the PI (i.e. the greater the impedance to blood flow). Importantly, in both the uterine and internal carotid arteries, the greatest reductions in PI with HRT have been observed in those patients with the longest intervals after menopause who have the highest pre-treatment values. If a change in arterial tone is an important mediator in arterial disease protection afforded by HRT, then patients who are many years postmenopausal will derive benefits. This is what some epidemiological studies have reported, and substantial benefits in terms of a reduction in arterial disease risk have been observed in women in their middle 70s.

It is not known whether the change in arterial tone with HRT, as assessed through measurements of the PI, is due to a locally acting mechanism (see Question 3.62), or whether it is a secondary phenomenon which follows a change in cardiac function. Despite these uncertainties, it is clear that oestradiol lack and replacement significantly influence arterial tone.

4.35 Will the addition of a progestogen negate the benefits of oestrogens on arterial disease risk?

This is not known. It is clear that progestogens partially antagonize the potential benefits of oestrogens on both lipid and lipoprotein metabolism, and also upon the arterial flow velocity waveform.

Broadly speaking, progestogens can be divided into those which are derivatives of progesterone (medroxyprogesterone acetate, MPA; dydrogesterone) or of testosterone (norethisterone; norgestrel). It has been recognized for many years that the latter group antagonize oestrogen benefits on lipids and lipoproteins, and increase total and LDL-cholesterol and reduce HDL-cholesterol. It was believed that these effects were due as much if not more to the androgenic rather than to the progestogenic potency of these synthetic steroids. For this reason, the lowest effective dose of norethisterone and norgestrel required for endometrial protection should be administered (see Questions 6.35 and 6.36. However, more recent data indicate that MPA also causes potentially undesirable lipid effects. In a 3-month prospective study of postmenopausal women taking oral oestradiol 2 mg/day the addition of MPA, 10 mg/day, reduced HDL-cholesterol by approx. 8% and HDL$_2$-cholesterol by as much as 18% (Fig. 4.9). This effect of a progesterone-derivative on lipid and lipoprotein metabolism does not appear to be class-specific because the other widely prescribed progesterone derivative, dydrogesterone, appears to cause little, if any, lipid changes.

The presentation of the data in Figure 4.9 (redrawn from the original paper and not adapted) illustrates the differences in the plasma concentrations of various lipid and lipoprotein moieties between pre-treatment and the combined oestrogen/progestogen phase of therapy. What it does not show are the lipid and lipoprotein levels during the oestrogen-only phase of treatment. To determine these, sampling must be performed at least twice: once during the oestrogen-only phase and then repeated during the oestrogen/progestogen phase of treatment. The data shown in Figure 4.10 were derived from one of the very few studies in which serial sampling was performed. The oestrogen was administered continuously and the progestogen norethisterone was added for 10 days in each 28-day treatment cycle. The results shown in Figure 4.10 illustrate two important points. (1) The lipid/lipoprotein response will depend upon the oestrogen dose: thus, an increase in dose of oral oestradiol from 1 mg to 2 mg and then to 4 mg/day produced greater decreases in LDL-cholesterol. These were opposed by the addition of norethisterone, 1 mg/day, both during and immediately after the phase of progestogen addition, but were not present throughout the treatment cycle. (2) With all three oestrogen doses the values remained depressed well below baseline even during the phase of progestogen addition. When considered over the 28-day treatment cycle, the antagonistic effects of the addition of this progestogen at this low daily dose on LDL-cholesterol concentrations are small. It is to be remembered that the majority of data reporting HRT benefits on arterial disease risk were derived from studies of unopposed oestrogen given cyclically, for 21 out of 28 days. With the combined oestrogen/progestogen regimens widely prescribed today, the oestrogen is given alone for between 16 and 18 days each 28-day treatment cycle. Finally, one potential benefit of progestogens when added to oral oestrogens is often overlooked. As stated previously (see Question 4.34), oral oestrogens increase plasma triglyceride levels and this is potentially undesirable. Oral progestogens reduce triglyceride levels to below the pre-treatment range, a potentially beneficial effect. For all these reasons, we believe that it is most unlikely that progestogen addition will negate oestrogen benefits upon arterial disease risk.

Identical comments apply to the effects of progestogen addition with

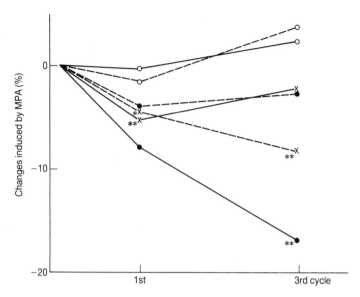

Fig. 4.9 Percentage change in mean total cholesterol and high-density lipoprotein cholesterol, its subfractions, and apolipoproteins following the sequential addition of 5 mg of medroxy-progesterone acetate (MPA) twice daily in 20 oestrogen-primed postmenopausal women. ×——×, total cholesterol; ×------×, HDL-cholesterol; ●——●, HDL$_2$-cholesterol; o——o, HDL$_3$-cholesterol; ●------●, apolipoprotein A1; o------o, apolipoprotein A2; * P< 0.05; ** P< 0.01. (From Ottosson UB, Johansson BG, von Schoultz BD 1985 American Journal of Obstetrics and Gynecology 151: 746–750. Reproduced with permission.)

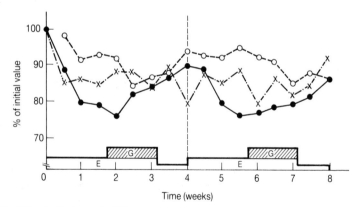

Fig. 4.10 Cyclic changes in LDL-cholesterol in relation to the oestrogen dose and the addition of norethisterone, 1 mg/day for 10 days. E and G indicate the oestrogen and progestogen components, respectively. ●——●, high oestrogen dose (4 mg/day); ×–·–×, medium oestrogen dose (2 mg/day); o------o, low oestrogen dose (1 mg/day). (From Jensen J, Nilas L, Christiansen C 1986 British Journal of Obstetrics and Gynaecology 93: 616–618. Reproduced with permission.)

respect to arterial flow velocity wave forms. The PI of the uterine artery is reduced by approximately 50% within 12 days of administering non-oral oestradiol (see Question 4.34 and Frontispiece). During the phase of progestogen addition, this reduction is partially antagonized from approximately 50% to approximately 35% below the pre-treatment value. The progestogenic effects are transient and have disappeared by the second week of oestrogen-only therapy in the next treatment cycle.

Few epidemiological studies of the effects of combined oestrogen/ progestogen therapy on arterial disease risk have been published. The data of Thompson et al on the effects of combined oestrogen/progestogen therapy on risk of MI and CVA have already been referred to (Table 4.1). The results from the Uppsala Health Study, from Sweden, have only been published in abstract form. They report that oestrogen-alone reduces arterial disease risk, and that this beneficial effect is not opposed by the addition of a progestogen.

Obviously, more data are urgently required with combination therapy. Because of the uncertainties over the effects of progestogen addition upon arterial disease risk and also because progestogens can cause symptomatic and psychological side-effects which may be severe, we believe that progestogens should only be prescribed if there is a clear indication (i.e. endometrial protection). We do not routinely add progestogens to the oestrogen in hysterectomized women (see Question 8.40).

4.36 Who will benefit most from the effects of HRT on arterial disease risk?

This is unknown. The lack of a suitable screening test for arterial disease (equivalent to bone density measurements in screening for osteoporosis) is discussed in Question 5.34.

The effects of HRT in sub-groups of women known to be at high-risk for arterial disease are presented in Question 5.36.

4.37 Will HRT be effective in reducing arterial disease risk if started many years after the menopause?

Scant data are available to answer this question. The available studies report that HRT is effective in women many years after menopause; substantial benefits have been reported in women in their middle-70s.

4.38 How long does HRT have to be prescribed before arterial benefits will be observed?

Again, only scant data are available. They indicate that some benefits are seen within 2 years of starting treatment.

4.39 Are the benefits of HRT upon arterial disease risk duration-dependent?

Based upon scarce data, the current belief is that extending the duration of therapy does not confer significantly greater benefits.

4.40 It is thought probable that HRT administered for 5 years soon after menopause will exert long-term benefits upon the skeleton: does the same apply for arterial disease risk?

No. It would appear that much of the beneficial effect of HRT on arterial disease risk is lost within a few years (perhaps 2 years) of stopping treatment.

4.41 Are the benefits of HRT on arterial disease risk dose-related?

Too few data are available to answer this question with any great confidence. The majority of the published studies refer to conjugated equine oestrogens, 0.625 mg/day, given cyclically. There is little information on 0.3 mg/day; the sparse data on 1.25 mg/day suggest that it is not twice as protective as 0.625 mg/day.

4.42 Will non-oral routes of oestrogen administration reduce arterial disease risk?

This is the 64 000-dollar question. We believe that they will, provided that a plasma oestradiol value similar to that achieved with conjugated equine oestrogens (0.625 mg/day) is achieved. The plasma oestradiol levels observed with various oral and non-oral preparations widely prescribed in the UK are considered in Questions 6.5 and 6.16.

5. When is HRT indicated?

The efficacy of oestrogens in relieving symptoms of vasomotor instability and genital tract atrophy has been established beyond doubt. These benefits, together with relief of psychological problems, can improve a woman's quality of life and this has been recognized for many years. Yet comparatively few women in the UK have received HRT. This may reflect a failure of recognition on the part of the medical profession that oestrogen deficiency symptoms can cause distress requiring treatment, coupled with anxieties about potential hazards of hormone therapy. More recently, it has become apparent that in asymptomatic, early postmenopausal women oestrogens can play a key role in the later prevention of osteoporotic fractures and arterial disease. These issues have attracted considerable media interest which has resulted in growing demands from the public for further information and treatment. Thus, we, as health care professionals, will be consulted by both symptomatic and asymptomatic patients.

In this chapter, we will endeavour firstly to clarify the indications for HRT with the aim of not only providing relief of distressing symptoms but of also targeting therapy towards those at greatest risk of later osteoporosis and arterial disease; and secondly to place the consequences of ovarian failure in a clinical setting.

DIAGNOSIS

It must be remembered that spontaneous 'natural' menopause can arise at any age. Our youngest patient was 18 years old. The following comments about the nature of typical climacteric complaints apply equally to all women, irrespective of age at menopause.

5.1 What are the typical symptoms of the climacteric and how should they be diagnosed?

In our experience, the presence of symptoms is a more reliable guide to accurate diagnosis than is endocrine investigations.

In the majority of patients, the history alone points to a clear diagnosis. The onset of typical hot flushes and night sweats and/or symptoms of lower genital tract atrophy, closely associated with oligomenorrhoea or amenorrhoea in a woman over age 40 years, is sufficient for a diagnosis of climacteric. In this age group, confirmatory laboratory investigations are not required. Because women can be shy about volunteering symptoms due to lower genital tract atrophy, direct enquiry must always be made. The precise date of the menopause (the last menstrual period) can only be documented with hindsight.

5.2 Of what other symptoms may the patient complain?

The clinical presentation, in our experience, may comprise any of the above complaints together with one or more of the following: tiredness, apathy, loss of interest, anxiety, irritability, mood swings, episodes of tearfulness, and poor concentration and memory. The latter may be so marked that the patient starts making lists of activities to be undertaken. We call this the 'jotter syndrome'. Not surprisingly, the patient may volunteer that she can no longer cope efficiently at home or at work. She may also complain of depression. The relationship between oestrogen deficiency and classic, endogenous depression has been referred to previously (see Question 3.28). Classic, endogenous depression does not appear to be related to the ovarian status and our belief is that the use of this term by peri- and postmenopausal women reflects their general lack of wellbeing.

Other symptoms, not related to the psychological status, include dry skin, dry hair, brittle nails, and musculo-skeletal discomfort or pains (see Question 3.36). Less commonly, patients may complain of formication (see Question 3.37), dry mouth and dry eyes.

All of the above symptoms are strongly suggestive of oestrogen deficiency. We stress that more often than not many will not be volunteered and therefore specific enquiry as to their presence must be made. Failure so to do may result in misdiagnosis and therefore inappropriate therapy, usually with hypnotics, sedatives and tranquillizers. The unfortunate woman may then be labelled 'neurotic' and may believe that she is going mad. *There is no substitute for an adequate history.* Biochemical investigations may not detect subtle reductions in oestradiol production and this is particularly true during the early climacteric when menstrual disturbances are minimal. In women with regular cycles, any of the above symptoms may be more pronounced premenstrually, and they may then be confused with premenstrual syndrome. The psychological problems of anxiety, irritability and mood swings can predominate in the premenstrual phase. Laboratory investigations are often unhelpful, especially in the early climacteric, because of the wide fluctuations in plasma FSH and oestradiol concentrations that occur at this time.

Plasma gonadotrophin levels may vary 4-fold during a 24-hour period in the early climacteric, from well within the premenopausal range to within the postmenopausal range. Some authors have maintained that an elevated FSH (over 15 iu/l) indicates that psychological symptoms will respond to oestrogen therapy. Others maintain that a therapeutic trial of HRT is more useful at resolving the dilemma of whether these disturbances, and particularly the psychological symptoms, are due to oestrogen deficiency or concurrent but coincidental domestic, social or economic stresses. Undoubtedly, this is a difficult area but an important one since symptoms resulting from stressful life events are best treated by psychiatrists, marriage guidance counsellors or social workers, not by oestrogen therapy.

5.3 How can the diagnosis of the climacteric be made in hysterectomized women with intact ovaries?

By using the same approach as detailed above. The lack of a uterus means that changes in menstruation, which are an important sign of early ovarian failure, are absent. Again, the presence of typical symptoms elicited by an appropriate history appears a more reliable diagnostic tool than reliance upon endocrine investigations, especially during the early climacteric.

PREMATURE MENOPAUSE

For reasons that will be discussed, women with premature menopause should be considered a 'high risk' group, particularly for the long-term consequences of ovarian failure. Premature menopause will now be considered in detail.

5.4 Does hysterectomy with ovarian conservation advance the age of failure in the retained ovaries?

There is a substantial literature that hysterectomy with ovarian conservation advances the age of failure in the retained ovaries. In our series, the age at which ovarian failure occurred was advanced by 4.1 years following hysterectomy. These data are shown in Figure 5.1. There was a highly significant correlation between the age at hysterectomy and the age at ovarian failure in the women who were 44 years or less at the time of ovarian failure. This implies a causal relationship. Thus, the development of typical climacteric symptoms soon after hysterectomy may not be coincidental, and these symptoms should not be overlooked especially in younger women.

The mechanism of action is unknown. It has been suggested that surgery may damage the blood supply to the ovary. Supportive evidence comes from reports that other forms of surgery, e.g. sterilization, have a similar effect. Alternatively, the uterus may release certain endocrine factors (as yet unidentified) which have a controlling influence upon ovarian function.

5.5 Apart from surgery, what are the other causes of premature menopause?

As indicated previously, spontaneous 'natural' menopause may occur at any age. It has been associated with chromosomal and also with certain auto-immune disorders.

An increasing number of women are being rendered menopausal at an early age through iatrogenic causes, notably radiotherapy and chemo-therapy. These may be administered to treat certain malignant diseases with a primary outside the pelvis, e.g. certain types of leukaemia, in which the ovary is a well-recognized site for metastatic disease. This group of patients will undoubtedly enlarge as treatment of the different diseases becomes more successful.

5.6 At what age is menopause considered to be 'premature'?

Most authorities would classify a premature menopause as occurring below age 40 years. Some would regard a menopause occurring before age 45 years as premature.

5.7 How may premature menopause be differentiated from other causes of secondary amenorrhoea?

The presence of typical oestrogen deficiency symptoms may suggest a diagnosis of ovarian failure. However, the converse does not apply because some women with premature menopause are asymptomatic. A diagnosis of premature menopause is usually confirmed by at least two and preferably three sets of gonadotrophin (and perhaps oestradiol) measurements within

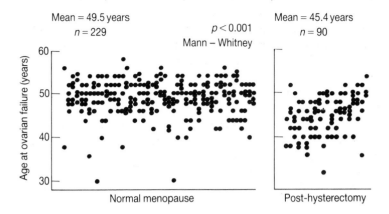

Fig. 5.1 Scattergrams of the age at ovarian failure in 229 women who had undergone spontaneous menopause and in 90 women after hysterectomy with bilateral ovarian conservation. n = numbers of patients. (From Siddle N, Sarrell P, Whitehead M I 1987 Fertility and Sterility 47: 94–100. Reproduced with permission.)

the postmenopausal range. In ovarian failure, FSH will be elevated and plasma oestradiol will be low. Repeated low or normal FSH values exclude premature menopause.

The only other condition in which FSH is elevated and plasma oestradiol is low on serial measurements is resistant ovary syndrome.

5.8 How may premature menopause be differentiated from resistant ovary syndrome?

Resistant ovary syndrome is rare and the aetiology is poorly understood. Oocytes are present within the ovary but they fail to respond to endogenous gonadotrophins and, in consequence, the plasma levels of the latter rise. Because oocyte maturation and ovulation does not occur, oestradiol is not produced. The cause of the syndrome (a gonadotrophin or ovarian abnormality) is not known, but the ovarian tissue usually contains an excess of mononuclear cells and it has been suggested that resistant ovary syndrome should be considered an autoimmune disorder.

The only reliable method of differentiating between premature menopause and resistant ovary syndrome is by ovarian biopsy. In practice, this is only indicated in women desiring fertility because there are reports of pregnancy following various hormonal manipulations in women with resistant ovary syndrome.

5.9 Why should we be concerned by premature menopause?

Some women with premature menopause will experience symptoms but others will not. Leaving aside these problems, women undergoing early loss of ovarian function who do not receive HRT are at an increase in risk of the early development of arterial disease and osteoporosis. An increase in risk of arterial disease following surgical oophorectomy was first reported more than 30 years ago; more recent data from a very large study are shown in Figure 5.2. This illustrates that the risk of arterial disease (cardiovascular disease) more than doubled in untreated women following premature menopause, but was not increased in those women receiving oral HRT after oophorectomy.

Premature menopause is also associated with the early development of osteoporosis. Women undergoing premature menopause around age 30 years will, 20 years later, have bone mass comparable to that in 70-year-old women who underwent natural menopause around age 50 years (Fig. 5.3).

5.10 How effectively is premature menopause being treated with HRT?

Sadly, the answer is poorly. A recent study showed that only 23% of women who had undergone hysterectomy and bilateral salpingo-oophorectomy before the age of 40 years had received HRT. Even among the treated group the duration of therapy was often inadequate.

It has recently been reported that in young women with ovarian failure due to successful treatment for leukaemia the consequences of oestrogen deficiency were associated with significant sexual difficulties, loss of self-esteem and feelings of loss of femininity. Many patients changed their social activities in consequence. The National Osteoporosis Society has also recently reported a disproportionately high number of women with premature menopause in the age group 60–65 years with osteoporotic fractures.

5.11 How long should HRT be continued after premature menopause?

There are no data available which have specifically addressed this question. In theory, it seems sensible to initiate therapy soon after the early menopause and to continue until the age of 50 years.

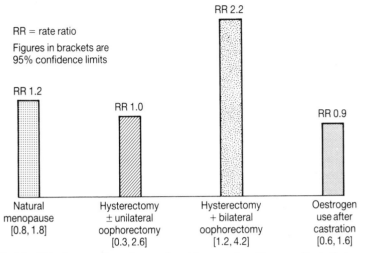

Fig 5.2 Risk of coronary heart disease, adjusted for age and smoking, according to the type of menopause (estimated from proportional analysis). (Adapted from Colditz et al 1987 New England Journal of Medicine 316: 1105–1110. Reproduced with permission.)

5.12 Can young women with premature menopause be treated with the oral contraceptive?

This is not known. The oestrogen dose in the oral contraceptive is a bone conserver. However, the long-term effects of oral contraceptive formulations in young women with functioning ovaries upon the later risk of arterial disease are controversial. Some studies have reported that long-term administration of the pill as a contraceptive may increase arterial disease risk. Thus, it is possible that HRT and oral contraceptive formulations have different effects upon arterial disease risk.

5.13 Should other groups of amenorrheic young women be treated as though they had premature menopause?

Yes. Our current understanding is that any prolonged period of amenorrhoea occurring during the reproductive era which is due to hypo-oestrogenism is likely to cause adverse skeletal and arterial changes. To date, the skeletal effects have been best documented in young amenorrhoeic women who exercise excessively and/or diet to extremes. Thus, this group includes sports 'freaks' and anorexics.

Additionally, any woman with a disease which has resulted in failure of the pituitary to produce endogenous gonadotrophins sufficient for ovarian stimulation should be made aware of the long-term consequences of prolonged oestrogen deprivation and offered replacement therapy.

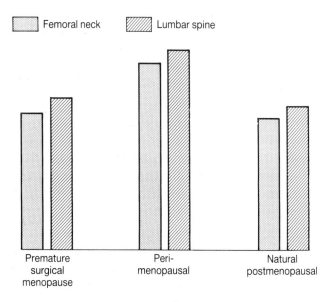

Premature surgical menopause
  Group with mean age 54 years and mean duration since oophorectomy 22 years
Perimenopausal
  Group with mean age 52 years
Natural postmenopausal
  Group with mean age 73 years and mean time since menopause 22 years

Fig. 5.3   Bone mineral density at two skeletal sites in perimenopausal women and women after natural and premature surgical menopause. (Adapted from Richelson et al 1984 New England Journal of Medicine 311: 1273–1275. Reproduced with permission.)

We will now return to discussing the indications for treatment in women undergoing menopause after age 45 years.

SYMPTOMATIC PATIENTS

5.14 What are the indications for treatment with HRT?

As in most other therapeutic areas, active therapy should be instituted when the physical or psychological wellbeing is adversely affected.

Symptoms may fall into one or more of the following categories: (a) vasomotor, (b) psychological/emotional, (c) atrophic (lower urogenital tract) and (d) collagen-related.

The decision to offer HRT will be based upon an assessment of the degree of distress caused by the symptoms weighed against the side-effects and risks of therapy. In addition, the known prophylactic benefits of HRT should be taken into account. Adequate discussion of these issues is essential. This may take time and may require two or more consultations. Because of pressure upon the doctor's time, other sources of information which will enable *the patient to make an informed decision* are often invaluable. These include reading material (books and leaflets), audio and video cassettes (which are available through the Amarant Trust—see page 224) and, most importantly, the experienced clinic or practice nurse who can provide counselling services.

The side-effects of the oestrogen and progestogen components of HRT are discussed in detail in Chapter 7. Very briefly, those that cause most problems are the re-establishment of regular withdrawal bleeding (which often deters women from starting therapy) and the progestogenic side-effects which are similar to premenstrual syndrome (anxiety, irritability, mood swings and breast discomfort). These may deter women from continuing with treatment. Thus, it is not surprising that patients who have undergone hysterectomy (who therefore will not bleed and do not need a progestogen) are more likely to opt for HRT and to stay on treatment even when their symptoms are relatively mild. For women who have not undergone hysterectomy the prospect of regular withdrawal bleeds is a deterrent to use of HRT, particularly when symptoms are mild. In general, women suffering symptoms of moderate or severe degrees find that the benefits of HRT outweigh the disadvantages.

5.15 Could the patient be offered a 'trial of therapy'?'

Yes. We believe that this is a greatly undervalued and underused option. It is most unlikely that any patient is going to suffer serious long-term consequences from a therapeutic trial lasting for three months. Because maximum benefits of oestrogens upon the relief of hot flushes may not be achieved for three months (Fig. 5.4), durations of treatment shorter than this are, we believe, insufficient if vasomotor disturbances are the principal symptoms.

5.16 When should therapy begin?

The ideal time to commence HRT is during the perimenopausal or early postmenopausal years.

However, it must be remembered that many premenopausal women with regular menstrual cycles suffer with hot flushes and night sweats (and sometimes other symptoms suggestive of declining ovarian function) for up to 7–10 days prior to menstruation. In some women this symptom-complex

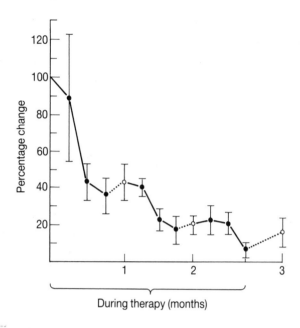

Fig. 5.4 Percentage change in mean (±SE) daily number of hot flushes with oestradiol (Estraderm®: Ciba-Geigy) 50 μg/day given cyclically. ● = on-treatment; ○ = off-treatment. (Adapted from Padwick M L, Endacott J, Whitehead M I 1985 American Journal of Obstetrics and Gynecology 152: 1085–1091. Reproduced with permission.)

may last for several years. We find that women in this group can be more difficult to treat successfully because of their fluctuating endogenous oestrogen levels. Thus, administration of a fixed daily dose of oestrogen in HRT may result in symptoms of oestrogen overdosage (bloatedness, breast tenderness) at the time in the cycle when ovarian activity is relatively normal. Use of combined oestrogen/progestogen HRT formulations in this group may provoke irregular bleeding because it is often difficult to synchronize exogenous progestogen with endogenous progesterone. This is especially difficult when the length of the menstrual cycle is variable. Thus, the use of conventional, combined HRT treatments in a premenopausal woman may involve a higher rate of side-effects and irregular vaginal bleeding than that seen in women commencing such therapy in the peri- or early postmenopausal years. An adverse experience at an early stage can deter future use of HRT and therefore a careful assessment of the severity of symptoms is required.

5.17 What are the disadvantages of starting HRT in pre-menopausal women?

As discussed above, it is more difficult to synchronize exogenous oestrogens and progestogens around a pre-existing endogenous, probably fluctuating, hormone milieu.

5.18 How may these problems be overcome?

Firstly, careful assessment should be made of the severity of symptoms and their likelihood of oestrogen responsiveness. Where symptoms fall into the milder categories simple explanation and reassurance may suffice.

If the symptoms are more troublesome then the provision of a *small oestrogen supplement* during the premenstrual week may be beneficial. For example, the use of the small oestradiol patch, 25 μg, or oral piperazine oestrone sulphate, 0.75 mg daily, during the premenstrual phase should be considered. While there are few prospective data on this strategy, our experience has been favourable. Such treatment may also help with menstrual migraine if the oestrogen supplement is continued for the first 2–3 days of menstruation when the migraine is often most severe. Before prescribing small oestrogen supplements we verify that endogenous progesterone production is adequate for endometrial protection by measuring the plasma progesterone level on the 7th day prior to menstruation.

An alternative strategy in the premenopausal woman with a regular cycle and premenstrual symptoms is to use a much higher oestrogen dose than that routinely administered in HRT. The aim of the higher dose is to suppress ovarian function and conventional HRT does not achieve this and therefore is not a contraceptive. Thus, continuous administration of transdermal oestradiol, 200 μg, or the use of oestradiol implants (usually 100 mg) will achieve benefits. In theory, high dose oral oestrogens will exert similar effects but, unlike transdermal and implant therapies, there are no reports on oral oestrogens. With high dose oestrogens exogenous progestogen has to be administered to protect against endometrial hyper-stimulation (see Question 6.37).

Such high doses of transdermal oestradiol are not usually required for effective symptom relief in perimenopausal and postmenopausal women.

5.19 Can perimenopausal and postmenopausal women experience surges of ovarian activity?

Yes. This is well documented and simply emphasizes that the decline in ovarian function is gradual and occurs over many years. The typical history in an untreated woman is that of troublesome symptoms lasting for some weeks/months which suddenly disappear usually for a period of 10–21 days, and which are then followed by typical premenstrual symptoms and by bleeding. If this occurs in a woman more than 12 months postmenopausal then appropriate investigations must be instituted.

Because conventional HRT does not suppress ovarian activity, similar surges in ovarian function occur in perimenopausal and postmenopausal women treated with combined oestrogen/progestogen HRT formulations. The bleeding may coincide with that induced by the exogenous progestogen, but it may occur at any time during the treatment cycle and is then defined as breakthrough bleeding. If one episode of breakthrough bleeding is preceded by typical prodromal symptoms of menstruation then we do not routinely offer endometrial biopsy. Two or more episodes of breakthrough bleeding demand appropriate investigation. (See Question 9.42).

5.20 Can we be sure that psychological/emotional symptoms are related to oestrogen deficiency?

This is frequently a difficult problem in pre-, peri- and postmenopausal women. It is impossible to be dogmatic, particularly when psychological symptoms are present in the absence of vasomotor symptoms. Careful history taking is important and adequate time should be allotted for discussion. It seems important not to attribute symptoms too quickly to a single cause, e.g. menopausal status or age. There are large individual differences in the aetiology of psychological symptoms and these have been extensively discussed (see Question 3.20).

Most authorities agree that hormonal investigations are of little value and therefore a therapeutic trial of HRT for 3 months should be considered (in the absence of absolute contraindications). The premenopausal woman with an intact uterus can be given an oestrogen supplement, or high dose oestrogen therapy with a progestogen as discussed above. Conventional, combined HRT regimens are suitable for perimenopausal and postmenopausal women who have not undergone hysterectomy. The value of progestogen addition in the hysterectomized woman is discussed in Question 8.40.

5.21 What about a 'trial of therapy' in a patient who has psychological symptoms which I do not think are related to the menopause?

The consequences of ovarian failure and oestrogen deficiency are multi-system and the relationship of many tissues to oestradiol is currently poorly understood (see Chapter 3). Because of the limited value of plasma oestradiol measurements in predicting the frequency and severity of certain symptoms, the 'acid test' with some symptoms is to prescribe a trial of therapy for 3 months and to monitor the response. If the symptom resolves with therapy it was due to oestrogen deficiency; the converse does not necessarily apply.

5.22 If there is an incomplete response to HRT what should be done?

Firstly, specific enquiry regarding compliance with therapy must be undertaken. Secondly, if partial relief was achieved then increasing the oestrogen dose and extending the trial for a further 3 months may produce greater benefits. This is particularly true if co-existing vasomotor symptoms were only partially alleviated during the initial trial. Failure to abolish flushes and sweats almost completely indicates a sub-optimal oestrogen dose. Thirdly, if no relief was achieved but concurrent vasomotor symptoms were abolished (which indicates that a therapeutic plasma oestradiol level was achieved), then the symptom in question cannot be due to oestrogen deficiency and alternative causes must be considered. Finally, if oral oestrogens were administered but the symptom in question was not improved and neither were concurrent hot flushes and night sweats, then an alternative route of administration should be considered. For reasons that are incompletely understood, a tiny percentage of women do not appear to absorb oestrogens well from the bowel and the failure of response of vasomotor symptoms to oral therapy confirms this. A non-oral route of administration should then be tried. Small bowel disease (especially if surgical resection has been performed) may exacerbate non-absorption of oral oestrogen.

In women who do not have concurrent vasomotor symptoms the only way to determine whether the plasma levels achieved with any route of administration are within the therapeutic range is by measurement of plasma oestradiol concentrations.

It is to be remembered that symptoms unequivocally due to oestrogen lack will be improved if adequate plasma oestradiol concentrations are achieved: failure of response in the presence of an adequate plasma level indicates that the symptom is not due to oestradiol deficiency. The menopause should not be regarded as a convenient coat peg upon which to hang all manner of weird and wonderful symptoms which can arise coincidentally during the climacteric years. HRT is not a panacea for all middle-aged ills, and some patients have expectations of HRT which are unrealistic.

ALTERNATIVES TO HRT

5.23 What alternative therapies are available for the management of vasomotor symptoms?

Few agents have been shown to be as effective as oestrogens in properly conducted placebo-controlled studies.

Progestogens, by themselves, have been shown to reduce the frequency of flushing episodes by 60–70%. For example, medroxyprogesterone acetate 10–20 mg or norethisterone 5–10 mg are considered useful, particularly in patients possessing contraindications to oestrogens (see Question 4.5 and Fig. 4.1).

Clonidine has been shown to be effective in placebo-controlled, cross-over studies of short duration. However, studies of longer duration have reported a failure of response of vasomotor symptoms to clonidine, and the two studies that compared clonidine with oestrogen therapy both reported that oestrogen was significantly better.

The effects of propranolol have been studied but with conflicting results.

Hypnotics, sedatives and tranquillizers have been widely prescribed but have not been shown capable of relieving vasomotor symptoms. Often such therapy only adds to the lethargy of which so many climacteric women complain.

There are anecdotal reports that hypnosis can be effective in achieving relief of vasomotor symptoms in some women. Various claims have been made for the beneficial effects of vitamin supplements such as vitamins B and E, and for evening primrose oil. Such claims may merely reflect the previously discussed placebo response.

5.24 What alternatives are available for the management of vaginal dryness and dyspareunia?

Alternatives to oestrogen creams are the traditional vaginal lubricants such as KY Jelly, etc. These agents may help the symptoms but, of course, will not reverse the atrophic changes. Many of our patients volunteer that while lubricants help with initial penetration, prolonged intercourse is impossible as the beneficial effects of the lubricant rapidly disappear.

ASYMPTOMATIC PATIENTS

5.25 When might HRT be indicated in asymptomatic climacteric and postmenopausal women?

The beneficial effects of HRT in terms of prophylaxis against osteoporosis and arterial disease have only recently become apparent. Therefore, the

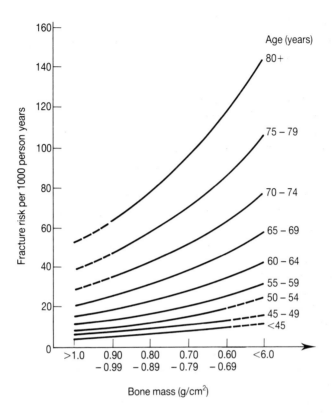

Fig. 5.5 The relationship between radial bone mass and subsequent fracture indicating an increased risk of fracture with declining bone mass in the stated age groups. (Hui S L, Slemenda C W, Johnston C 1988 Journal of Clinical Investigation 81: 1804–1809. Reproduced with permission.)

request from asymptomatic women for information about HRT is a relatively new development. The skeletal effects of oestrogen deficiency and oestrogen replacement have been extensively discussed in Chapters 3 and 4, respectively.

In summary, oestrogens prevent early postmenopausal bone loss and greatest benefits have been observed in women starting treatment soon after menopause, before significant bone is lost. However, oestrogens can also prevent bone loss when started many years after menopause. Oestrogens greatly reduce the risk of osteoporotic fracture when started in the early postmenopausal years but it is not clear whether similar benefits occur when they are first started many years after menopause. Bone density is significantly correlated with fracture risk (Fig. 5.5) and, therefore, stabilization of the skeleton in women with established disease by HRT should reduce the subsequent fracture rate. However, re-establishment of normal bone architecture cannot be achieved (see Fig. 4.4).

5.26 How should HRT be targeted?

Ideally, HRT should be targeted towards those women at greatest risk of osteoporosis and of arterial disease. Unfortunately, the reliable methods for screening for osteoporosis are not widely available and are expensive, and we have no reliable screening tool for arterial disease.

5.27 What screening methods are available to identify women at greatest risk of osteoporosis?

There are three possible methods of screening for those at greatest risk of osteoporosis:

1. Risk factor assessment charts
2. Bone densitometry measurements
3. Biochemical markers.

Two main factors determine a woman's susceptibility to postmenopausal osteoporosis: (a) the peak adult bone mass and (b) the subsequent rate of bone loss. Factors which appear to affect adult peak bone mass have been discussed (see Question 3.47). The primary cause of bone loss after menopause is loss of ovarian function.

5.28 What is the value of risk factor assessment charts in screening for osteoporosis?

Traditionally, risk factor charts (Table 3.2) have been used to make an assessment of an individual's risk of developing postmenopausal osteoporosis. These charts attempt to predict risk on the basis of factors which include genetic predisposition, physical characteristics, lifestyle, menstrual and obstetric history, and previous tobacco and alcohol use. While many of these factors may be associated with risk of osteoporosis in whole populations they are of little predictive value when applied to individuals. We have experience of women with significant risk factors (premature menopause, a strong family history of osteoporosis, a sedentary lifestyle, and heavy cigarette and alcohol consumption) who have normal bone density in the spine and the hip 5 years after menopause. Conversely, we have seen apparently healthy women who have menstruated until the late 50s, who have no family history of osteoporosis, who are of high parity, and who have never used tobacco or alcohol but in whom early spinal and hip osteoporosis has been diagnosed by bone density measurements within 18 months of menopause.

Thus, the value of risk factors in an individual woman can be low, and the doctor and patient must be aware of these limitations. However, for many doctors and most patients the risk factor chart is the only method currently available.

5.29 What is the value of bone densitometry measurements in screening for osteoporosis?

At present, identifying women most at risk of later osteoporosis is best achieved by bone densitometry measurements. Unfortunately, facilities for measuring bone density fall far short of the need. A list of useful addresses where bone density measurements are performed is given in Appendix 1.

It is important to appreciate that reliable methodologies for bone density measurements are a relatively recent introduction. Techniques for the wrist, spine and hip were introduced during the late 1970s, early 1980s and late 1980s, respectively. Indeed, the hip methodology is so new that only one study has prospectively reported the effects of HRT at this site (see Fig. 4.7), and the majority of the hip data currently available are cross-sectional. Because the natural history of osteoporosis may extend over a period as long as 30 years, it is not surprising that this has been studied cross-sectionally, not longitudinally, and our knowledge of the relative importance of certain factors in predicting this disease remains incomplete.

5.30 What are the limitations of bone density measurements?

These will be discussed under the following headings:

(a) *How reliable is a bone density measurement at predicting future osteoporosis?*

Bone density is a strong predictor of fracture risk (see Fig. 5.5). From cross-sectional studies, it is clear that the best predictor of bone density at age 70 years is bone density at age 50 years. Thus, bone density measurements performed around natural menopause will assist in the identification of women at high risk for later osteoporosis.

(b) *Does it matter which anatomical site is measured?*

Yes. Wrist measurements are usually performed using single or dual photon absorptiometry (SPA or DPA). It is relatively easy to obtain good accuracy with both. Spinal bone density measurements have been performed using quantitative computed tomography (QCT) and also DPA. The former involves a higher radiation exposure than the latter. Good accuracy, which is essential in a screening programme, is more difficult to obtain with spinal DPA and QCT than with wrist SPA or DPA measurements. Until very recently, only DPA could be used to measure hip bone density.

SPA and DPA possess the disadvantage of using a radioactive source which is subject to decay and this, potentially, is an important source of error in the measurement (see below). The recent introduction of dual energy X-ray absorptiometry (DEXA) which does not rely on radioactive sources should overcome this problem. Preliminary data indicate that DEXA achieves high accuracy in both the spine and hip.

Wrist bone density measurements do not correlate well with those in the much more clinically relevant sites of the spine and hip. Correlations between forearm and spinal measurements in early postmenopausal women are shown in Table 5.1. We have seen patients with normal wrist bone density who have early spinal osteoporosis. Similarly, the correlation between spine and hip bone density is also poor. Thus, to determine the later risk of fracture at a given anatomical site (wrist, spine or hip), site-specific measurements appear essential. The later risk of hip fracture cannot be determined from a bone density measurement performed at the wrist.

(c) *What are the pitfalls in interpreting bone density measurements?*
Bone density measurements are expressed in absolute values for that anatomical site in a given individual. If the accuracy of the particular machine is sub-optimal then the measurements are likely to be unreliable and of no value. Good units undertaking bone density measurements using DPA (particularly at the spine) will also perform in-vitro and in-vivo measurements to determine accuracy as part of a continuing quality control programme. Similar comments apply to DEXA.

The values from an individual are compared to a 'normal' range to determine whether that individual patient has high, normal or low bone density. The 'normal' range should have been constructed from data obtained from women similar to the individual patient. It is inappropriate to compare the results from a black woman with a normal range derived from a white population and vice versa. Ideally, the normal range should have been established using the same machine and from measurements performed in local patients. Again, comparing the results from a patient in a provincial town in the United Kingdom with a 'normal' range established in women in North America may be inappropriate.

5.31 When should bone density measurements be performed?

Assessment of bone density is best made at or around the time of the

Table 5.1. Interrelations of the various bone mass measurements (BD = bone density; BMC = bone mineral content; TBCa = total body calcium)

	Vertebral BMC	Forearm trabecular BMC	Forearm integral BD	Forearm cortical BD
Forearm trabecular BMC	0.53			
Forearm integral BD	0.51	0.72		
Forearm cortical BD	0.40	0.55	0.70	
TBCa	0.54	0.64	0.84	0.73

P < 0.001. Adapted from Stevenson J C, Banks L M, Spinks T J et al 1987 Journal of Clinical Investigation 80: 258–262.

menopause. Assuming a normal rate of postmenopausal bone loss the bone mass measurement at the time of the menopause can be used to predict the subsequent degree of risk of osteoporosis. It is currently believed that a woman with a low bone mass at menopause will have a high likelihood of osteoporosis whereas a woman with a high bone mass at menopause is unlikely to develop this disease. Women who lie between these extremes may need repeat measurements of bone density before a final decision can be made about the risk of later osteoporosis.

Therefore, ideally, all women should have bone density measurements at the time of the menopause to assess whether they have high, average or low bone mass. In practice, this is very difficult since access to facilities is very restricted, particularly within the National Health Service. The private sector is increasingly offering bone density measurements. It is hoped that the current costs of spine and hip measurements (which start at around £150, privately) will be reduced as DEXA machines become more widely available. DEXA possesses the great advantage of a much shorter scanning time than QCT and DPA and therefore more patients can be screened per unit time. The radiation exposure with DEXA is less than that of a conventional chest X-ray.

We believe that much greater efforts are required to identify and treat women with a premature menopause who are at greatest risk. Perhaps bone density measurements should be reserved for this group of women and also those who lack menopausal symptoms but who would take HRT if they were shown to be at an increased risk for later osteoporosis. There is a growing public awareness of the problems of osteoporosis but uptake of health education resources is greatest in the financially and educationally advantaged sectors of society. If all women at risk are to be identified systematic health education and screening methods will be required.

It is not known whether screening around menopause and targeting HRT at high-risk women will be cost-effective. Pilot studies to answer this question have been started in the United Kingdom but the results may not be available for some years.

5.32 Is it worthwhile offering bone density measurements to women some years past the menopause?

Probably, yes. For reasons discussed previously, stabilization of the rate of bone loss in women with early osteoporosis should reduce the risk of fracture as compared to a similar untreated group. Not uncommonly, early osteoporosis may have already compromised the skeleton sufficiently for fracture to occur. Women with early osteoporotic fractures (Colles' fracture of the wrist; first vertebral crush fracture) should be regarded as being at higher risk for further fracture and considered for bone density measurements. However, early but significant bone loss may be clinically 'silent'. Despite their limitations, we believe that women with one or more significant risk factors (particularly the previously untreated woman with premature menopause) should be made aware that they may be at an increase in risk for later osteoporosis, and that bone density measurements should be discussed with them.

It is not known whether routine screening of asymptomatic women 10–15 years after menopause will be cost-effective.

5.33 What is the value of biochemical markers in screening for osteoporosis?

It has been suggested that a combination of simple biochemical tests can be used to diagnose those women suffering rapid bone loss after the menopause. Using various blood and urine tests, performed once early in the postmenopause, a 90% accuracy was claimed. However, it is not clear whether such information is helpful in deciding who to treat with HRT unless the bone density is also known. A high rate of bone loss may be irrelevant to future fracture risk if the bone density is high. Much further work is required before this method can be recommended.

5.34 What alternatives to HRT are available for prophylaxis against osteoporosis?

Alternative therapeutic agents include calcitonin and the bisphosphonates. Both these agents, like oestrogen, are antiresorptive. They are being actively researched and both show potential as alternatives to oestrogen for women who either cannot, or do not wish to, take HRT.

Sodium fluoride has been suggested as an alternative but many doubts remain as to its efficacy and safety. The recently presented data from the large placebo-controlled study performed in North America showed that while sodium fluoride increased bone density it was associated with an increased incidence of hip fracture. We believe that the use of sodium fluoride should be restricted to specialized centres performing research with this agent.

The value of calcium supplementation in early postmenopausal women has been discussed previously (see Question 4.28).

5.35 Can we identify women at greatest risk of later arterial disease?

Not really. Most work on risk factors for arterial disease has been performed in men, and the available data in women are sparse. There is no single test or set of tests in screening for arterial disease which mirrors the role of bone density measurements in screening for osteoporosis.

Some major risk factors are unalterable such as genetic predisposition and increasing age. The modifiable major risk factors are smoking, hypertension, and those hyperlipidaemias which increase the plasma levels of low density lipoprotein (LDL)-cholesterol and thereby total cholesterol, increase triglycerides and reduce high density lipoprotein (HDL)-cholesterol values. All these are of paramount importance. Other risk factors include diabetes, obesity, lack of exercise, an abnormal fibrinolytic/coagulation profile, stress, etc.

In the absence of a well-defined screening test, the commonsense approach is the only alternative. Where appropriate, the above factors should be treated by drugs (antihypertensives, lipid-lowering agents, insulin or oral hypoglycaemics), or by advice to change the lifestyle to eliminate or reduce the risk factor.

5.36 Is there an upper age limit for initiating HRT to reduce arterial disease risk?

In theory, there is no upper age limit for initiating HRT. Indeed, one study

Table 5.2 Acute MI mortality per 1000.

		Never	Ever	p value
Acute MI		4.8	2.6	0.007
Previous MI/angina	No	3.8	2.0	< 0.05
	Yes	10.7	5.2	< 0.05
Previous Hypertension	No	3.6	2.0	< 0.05
	Yes	6.4	3.0	< 0.05
Smoking	Never	4.9	2.0	< 0.05
	Ever	4.7	4.1	n.s.

Adapted from Henderson B E et al 1986 American Journal of Obstetrics and Gynecology 154 (1): 181–186. Reproduced with permission.

has reported substantial benefits with respect to arterial disease reduction in a group of women with a median age of 73 years.

5.37 What about the effects of HRT in sub-groups at high risk for arterial disease?

As discussed in Chapter 4, there is considerable evidence that oestrogens reduce arterial disease risk. It is again stressed that the majority of these data apply to therapy with oestrogen prescribed by itself, not combined with a progestogen.

At least three studies have determined the effects of oestrogen-only therapy in sub-groups of women possessing risk factors for arterial disease; data from one of these studies are reproduced in Table 5.2. As a group, women with a previous history of myocardial infarction (MI) or angina were at an increased risk from further, fatal MI. This is not surprising. However, when sub-divided into never or ever-users of postmenopausal oestrogen therapy, significant differences were observed between these sub-groups. Thus, ever-users of oestrogens had less than one half the risk of further but fatal MI as compared to non-users. Identical comments apply to the risk of fatal MI associated with a history of hypertension, with the never-users having a risk more than twice that of ever-users of HRT. Thus, oestrogen use in postmenopausal women with a history of MI, angina or hypertension more than halved the risk of later death from MI as compared to no use.

As discussed in Chapter 4, it has been argued that all the data upon arterial disease risk in postmenopausal oestrogen users are confounded by a selection bias. While this may have occurred in the general study population (which may have possessed less risk factors than the non-users), the results in Table 5.2 apply to women with known risk factors. Interestingly, the observed protective effect in these high-risk patients apparently afforded by oestrogen therapy was approximately a 50% reduction in fatal MI, which is similar to the protective effect observed in the general study population.

By including these results here we are being deliberately provocative. However, the data argue that postmenopausal oestrogen use is protective against fatal MI in women with a history of MI, angina or hypertension. If further supportive evidence becomes available, then it would not be unreasonable to argue that these high-risk groups should be considered for postmenopausal oestrogen therapy.

6. Types of HRT available

The principal hormones used in HRT are oestrogen and progestogen. The number and types of preparations have increased with new developments during the last 10 years. For each hormone, the type of preparation available, the route of administration, the dosage and the prescribing schedule need to be considered.

OESTROGENS

6.1 What types of oestrogen are available?

There are two types: synthetic and natural.

Synthetic oestrogens give rise to substances in the plasma which have potent oestrogenic activity but which are structurally dissimilar to the oestrogens produced by the ovary. Examples include ethinyl oestradiol, mestranol and stilboestrol. There are concerns about the use of synthetic oestrogens in HRT (see Question 6.2).

The natural oestrogens include oestradiol, oestrone and oestriol; many are synthesised. These are substances which, regardless of the method of manufacture/extraction, give rise in plasma to oestrogens which are identical to those produced by the premenopausal ovary. Conjugated equine oestrogens contain about 50–65% of oestrone sulphate and the remainder is made up of equine oestrogens, primarily equilin sulphate. Although, strictly speaking, they are not natural to humans these oestrogens behave in a similar manner and are generally classified as natural.

The natural oestrogens that are available for use in HRT, the route of administration and the principal plasma product are shown in Table 6.1. Systemic absorption with certain vaginal formulations is so low that accurate determination of the principal plasma product is not possible.

Table 6.1 Natural oestrogens, classified by route of administration, name (proprietary, composition and principal plasma product

Route	Proprietary name	Generic name	Principal plasma product
Oral	Premarin®	Conjugated equine oestrogen (60% approx. oestrone sulphate)	Oestrone
	Progynova®	Oestradiol valerate	Oestrone
	Harmogen®	Piperazine oestrone sulphate	Oestrone
	Hormonin®	Oestriol/oestrone/ oestradiol	Oestrone
	Ovestin®	Oestriol	Oestriol
Transdermal	Estraderm®	Oestradiol	Oestradiol
Subcutaneous		Oestradiol	Oestradiol
Vaginal	Premarin®	Conjugated equine oestrogens	Oestrone
	Ovestin®	Oestriol	?
	Orthogynest®	Oestriol	?
	Vagifem®	Oestradiol	?

6.2 Why are natural oestrogens preferable to synthetic oestrogens?

Synthetic oestrogens, as prescribed in the oral contraceptive, exert a pharmacological effect (suppression of ovulation). To achieve this, they possess greater potency than the natural oestrogens which are used in HRT and which, for the most part, achieve physiological levels of plasma oestradiol and/or oestrone.

Various parameters have been used in an attempt to quantify the relative potency of the synthetic and natural oestrogen preparations. One of the major concerns with the oral contraceptive has been the risk of venous thrombotic disease believed due to the oestrogen component. Synthetic oestrogens can alter, within the liver, the production rates of various factors involved in fibrinolysis/coagulation. Thus, the relative potencies of various natural and synthetic oestrogens on certain hepatic markers and other end-organs have been determined.

Table 6.2 Relative potency estimated according to four specific parameters of oestrogenicity

Oestrogen preparation	Serum FSH	Serum CBG-BC	Serum SHBG-BC	Renin substrate
Piperazine oestrone sulphate	1.0	1.0	1.0	1.0
Micronized oestradiol	1.3	1.9	1.0	0.7
Conjugated oestrogens	1.4	2.5	3.2	3.5
Diethylstilboestrol	3.8	70	28	13
Ethinyl oestradiol	(80–200)*	(1000)*	614	232

*Estimate in the absence of parallelism

(From Mashchak C A et al 1982 American Journal of Obstetrics and Gynecology 144: 511–518. Reproduced with permission.)

The data from one such study are shown in Table 6.2, and are expressed in milligram-equivalents of piperazine oestrone sulphate. This was ascribed a relative potency of 1.0 in each of the four systems studied: three of these were hepatic markers [induction of renin substrate, cortisol binding globulin (CBG) and sex hormone binding globulin (SHBG)], and the fourth marker was suppression of plasma follicle stimulating hormone (FSH). Micronised oestradiol had a similar potency to piperazine oestrone sulphate in all of the four systems. Conjugated equine oestrogens were slightly more potent ($\times$ 2.5– $\times$ 3.5) with respect to the hepatic markers. Both synthetic oestrogens, diethylstilboestrol and ethinyl oestradiol showed much enhanced hepatic potency. Ethinyl oestradiol was 230–1000 times more potent with respect to the hepatic markers studied and 80–200 times more potent than piperazine oestrone sulphate in suppressing FSH. This explains why this synthetic preparation is so effective as a contraceptive. However, the enhanced hepatic effects of ethinyl oestradiol are undesirable, especially in postmenopausal women. It is likely that similar differences in potency between the synthetic and natural oestrogens occur with respect to fibrinolytic and coagulation factors, and significant changes in these may be converted into clinical disease especially in older women. Coagulation research groups who have examined both synthetic and natural oestrogens have reported that the severity and spectrum of change is greater with the synthetic forms.

The greater potency of ethinyl oestradiol is due to the presence of an ethinyl group in the configuration at the C–17 position of the oestradiol molecule. This means that degradation by the principal, intracellular enzymes, the 17 β dehydrogenases, cannot occur. These enzymes cannot oxidize the hydroxyl group because of the covalent bond on carbon 17. As a result ethinyl oestradiol, which is readily absorbed from the gut and which passes unchanged via the portal system into the liver, passes into hepatocytes and following receptor binding has a prolonged, intracellular retention span. Additionally, the half-life of ethinyl oestradiol is approximately 7 hours and it does not bind to SHBG. In contrast, oestradiol 17 β which is the principal biologically active natural oestrogen is extensively bound to SHBG and only a small percentage is 'free' and physiologically active: the half life of oestradiol 17 β is approximately 90 minutes. All these differences contribute to the enhanced potency of ethinyl oestradiol.

Conjugated equine oestrogens are the most widely prescribed HRT preparation in Great Britain and the USA. As previously stated the main component is oestrone sulphate which accounts for about 50–65%. The remainder is made up of equine oestrogens which are structurally very similar to natural oestrogens except that the beta ring of the steroid molecule has an unsaturated bond. Also, they occur as 17 β and 17 α isomers. Because of these structural differences from oestradiol 17 β they, too, are likely to be more resistant to enzymatic metabolism within the liver and other target organs. This may explain the slightly greater potency of this preparation over the other oestradiol and oestrone preparations with respect to hepatic effects shown in Table 6.2. However, these differences are small and to all intents and purposes they are considered part of the natural oestrogen group.

6.3 What routes are available for oestrogen administration?

Although there are many potential routes of administration, (buccal, sublingual, intra-muscular), in practice only four are in common use in the UK: oral; transdermal (patch); subcutaneous (implant) and intra-vaginal. The principal question when deciding upon the route of administration to be used is whether it should be oral or non-oral.

6.4 What are the differences between the oral and non-oral routes of oestrogen administration?

The major difference between oral and non-oral administration is the avoidance of the gastrointestinal tract and 'first pass' effect on the liver with the non-oral route. Oral administration of oestrogen results in an initial rapid conversion of oestradiol to oestrone in the gut mucosa. Thus, regardless of the type of oestrogen prescribed orally (i.e. an oestradiol or an oestrone preparation) all are largely absorbed into the portal venous system as oestrone (see Table 6.1). Thus, oral oestradiol valerate (Progynova ®; Schering) and piperazine oestrone sulphate (Harmogen ®; Abbott) give very similar if not identical plasma products. After absorption, the oestrogens pass via the portal vein to the liver where they are further metabolized and inactivated. It has been estimated that 30–90% of the administered dose may be inactivated by the liver before the systemic circulation is reached.

These effects have a number of consequences. First, oestrone will be the dominant circulating oestrogen in the plasma. Second, the administered dose of oestrogen has to be correspondingly higher than that given by the non-oral route to achieve the same therapeutic plasma levels. Third, there is a wide inter-patient variation in the rate of absorption from the bowel and thus, different individuals may achieve dissimilar plasma levels despite the same oral dose. There is also the potential that the concurrent use of other drugs, such as phenobarbitone and carbamazepine which within the liver induce enzymes which metabolise oestrogens, may render standard doses of oral oestrogens ineffective. Fourth, there is the potential that in their passage through the liver orally administered oestrogens may influence other hepatic enzyme systems. As the liver is the principal site of synthesis of various plasma proteins and globulins including clotting factors, SHBG and renin substrate, it is possible that the production of these substances may be influenced more by oral than non-oral oestrogens. As already discussed, the extent of these effects will depend with the oral route on the potency of the various oestrogens prescribed, and they are also considered further below (Question 6.6).

Conjugated equine oestrogens at high dose have been shown to increase the production of renin substrate. However, the type of renin substrate so induced is not the one normally associated with hypertension and the clinical relevance of this change is unclear. Certainly in a number of placebo-controlled studies, oral conjugated equine oestrogens have not been associated with an increase in systolic or diastolic blood pressure. Nevertheless, it may well be advisable to avoid oral oestrogens in women who are considered susceptible to hypertension. The relationships between oral oestrogens and hypertension are considered further in Question 9.48.

The same situation applies to venous thrombotic disease. Although the production of certain clotting factors may be increased by oral oestrogens, the clinical significance of this is not clear. Oral natural oestrogens have not been convincingly shown to lead to an increase in risk of venous thrombotic disease in postmenopausal women (see also Question 8.7).

Not all the effects of the 'first pass' metabolism seen with oral oestrogens are considered adverse. Oestrogens have an effect on lipid and lipoprotein metabolism which is thought to be one of the major reasons whereby they reduce cardiovascular disease risk. The changes, a lowering of total cholesterol and low-density lipoprotein cholesterol and an increase in high-density lipoprotein cholesterol, appear dose-related. These aspects were discussed in Question 4.33.

It must be emphasized that although there are some potential drawbacks with oral therapy (hypertension, venous thrombotic disease), these are by and large unconfirmed whereas the long-term benefits of this route of administration are well proven. The vast majority of the long-term data on the benefits and safety of HRT relate to oral oestrogens, mainly conjugated equine oestrogens.

Non-oral oestrogens, whether patches or implants, avoid the first pass effect on the liver. Consequently, oestradiol can be preferentially delivered directly into the systemic circulation. The large, non-physiological increases in plasma oestrone values (which are of unknown clinical relevance) which are seen with oral therapy do not occur with these non-oral routes. To achieve similar plasma concentrations of the most biologically active natural oestrogen, oestradiol, as compared to the oral route, the administered dose can be reduced because degradation and inactivation does not occur before the systemic circulation is reached. Thus, oral oestrogens are administered in milligrams whereas transdermal oestrogens are given in micrograms. Because of the inter-patient variation in degradation and metabolism after reaching the systemic circulation varying plasma oestradiol values are also seen with non-oral delivery systems.

6.5 What are the plasma oestradiol values achieved with oral and non-oral routes of administration?

It is stressed that because of the marked inter-patient variation in absorption and metabolism, wide ranges in values occur with any preparation and route.

The mean values achieved with conjugated equine oestrogens 0.625 mg/day and 1.25 mg/day, and with transdermal oestradiol 50 μg/day and 100 μg/day are shown in Figure 6.1. For comparison, the plasma oestradiol values observed during the normal menstrual cycle are also shown. In our assay system, the lower and higher doses of these two preparations provide similar mean values: with the lower doses, the values are approximately 200 pmol/l (equivalent to day 6 to day 8 of the cycle) and with the higher doses are approximately 360 pmol/l (equivalent to day 8 to day 10 of the menstrual cycle). We believe it important to bear these comparisons constantly in mind. These oral and non-oral preparations do not even achieve the values within the premenopausal, peri-ovulatory phase range (approximately 1000 pmol/l), the time of maximal oestradiol production in the non-pregnant woman. Regularly menstruating women are exposed to values higher than those achieved with these HRT preparations each month from menarche to menopause. If HRT is as dangerous as some contend then no woman would live to experience menopause!

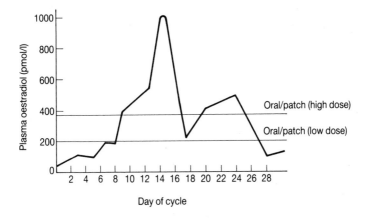

Figure 6.1 Plasma oestradiol levels (pmol/1) achieved by conjugated equine oestrogens, 0.625 mg/day or transdermal oestradiol 50 μg/day [(oral/patch (low dose)] or by conjugated equine oestrogens 1.25 mg/day or transdermal oestradiol 100 μg/day [(oral/patch (high dose)] as compared to levels during the normal, premenopausal menstrual cycle. Day 1 = first day of menstruation.

6.6 Do only oral oestrogens affect hepatic metabolism?

No. This belief has arisen largely, we believe, because of a mis-interpretation.

Comparisons of the effects of oral and non-oral oestrogens on various hepatic markers such as renin substrate and sex hormone binding globulin (SHBG) are shown in Figure 6.2. These markers were increased with oral but not with non-oral therapies. Thus, one explanation is that only oral oestrogens impact upon hepatic markers. Such an explanation, however, ignores two physiological processes. Firstly, the entire circulating blood volume is cleared through the liver approximately every 5 minutes and secondly, women utilize oestrogens efficiently through entero-hepatic recycling or 'second pass' metabolism. This is the process whereby oestrogens, after hepatic metabolism, are excreted in the bile and then reabsorbed in the lower part of the small bowel passing eventually back to the liver. Interference with entero-hepatic recycling may well be the mechanism whereby antibiotics cause breakthrough bleeding even in women receiving non-oral oestrogen preparations (see Question 9.35).

Thus, all oestrogens circulating in the plasma, regardless of the initial route of administration, will eventually pass through the liver and may be recycled. Consequently, if given for sufficient time, both oral and non-oral oestrogens may cause similar hepatic effects. This is borne out by the lipid and lipoprotein changes seen with the oral and non-oral routes (see

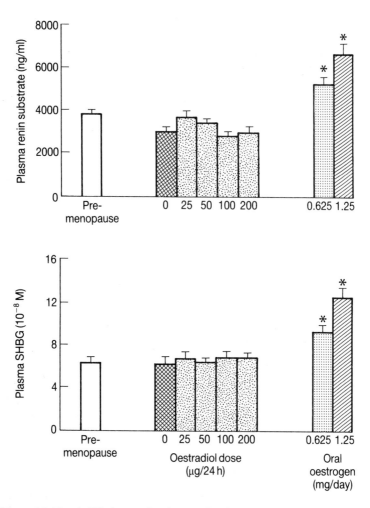

Figure 6.2 Mean (± SE) plasma renin substrate and sex hormone binding globulin (SHBG) in premenopausal women ☐, untreated postmenopausal women ▨, and during therapy (shaded boxes) with various doses of transdermal oestradiol and oral conjugated equine oestrogens (*significantly different from the baseline levels in postmenopausal women). (Adapted from Chetkowski R J, Meldrum D R, Steingold K A et al 1986 New England Journal of Medicine 314: 1615–1620. Reproduced with permission.)

Question 4.33). It was suggested that non-oral oestrogens would not have the beneficial effects on lipid metabolism seen with oral therapy. While the latter may give marginally greater effects, there are several reports that intramuscular, percutaneous and subcutaneous oestrogens have a similar impact on lipid metabolism when compared to the oral route. The most striking difference is that oral oestrogens increase triglycerides but non-oral oestrogens do not.

What, then, is the explanation for this difference and also the differences in effect between the oral and non-oral routes shown in Figure 6.2? We believe that the most likely explanation is that the changes seen with oral therapy are due not so much to the route of administration but more to the manner of delivery of the steroid, as a 'bolus'. Within 3–6 hours of administration of an oral oestrogen, the plasma levels of the principal metabolite of oestradiol have increased dramatically. Non-oral routes do not deliver the oestrogen, each day, as a bolus. We believe that it is the bolus which produces pharmacological effects and this would explain the increase in renin substrate and SHBG with oral oestrogens. A pharmacological action of oral oestrogens whereby hepatic secretion of very low density lipoproteins (VLDL) was increased would explain the elevated triglyceride levels seen with oral therapy.

6.7 Is the oral 'bolus' advantageous or disadvantageous?

This depends upon which hepatic marker is being considered. A lowering in low-density lipoprotein cholesterol would be seen as beneficial but a rise in triglyceride is not (see Question 4.33).

One set of hepatic markers about which little is known are the fibrinolytic/coagulation factors, and whether they are influenced in a similar or dissimilar manner by the oral and non-oral routes. Few data are available to draw meaningful conclusions, but one study has suggested that non-oral oestrogens do not change antithrombin III whereas oral oestrogens cause small, but definite, potentially adverse changes.

6.8 How should I decide which route to use?

The advantages and disadvantages of the main routes of administration are outlined in Table 6.3 and are discussed in detail in the next sections. As already stated, the vast majority of the long-term data on the benefits and safety of HRT relate to oral oestrogens. No such data are yet available for non-oral routes of administration but, as they achieve comparable plasma levels and have similar therapeutic effects to oral oestrogens, we think it reasonable to assume that they will have similar long-term benefits and risks.

Thus, in clinical practice, the choice of route of administration devolves upon patient and clinician preference in the majority of patients. Oral therapy need only be avoided in those women considered to be susceptible to the hepatic effects that we have already discussed, e.g. those with labile

Table 6.3 Routes of administration: Advantages and disadvantages

Route	Advantages	Disadvantages
Oral	Easy to administer Easy to stop Short half-life Hepatic effects	Compliance not guaranteed Nausea and dyspepsia ?Physiological Hepatic effects
Transdermal	Easy to administer Easy to stop Short half-life Non-oral but hepatic effects	Compliance not guaranteed Skin reactions Progestogen has to be given orally
Implants	Compliance guaranteed Testosterone can be added	Administration requires minor surgery Long carry-over effect Difficult to stop Progestogen has to be given orally Tachyphylaxis

blood pressure, hypertriglyceridaemia or a previous history of venous thromboembolism. In addition, women with chronic gastrointestinal diseases (especially of the small bowel) are likely to benefit from the non-oral route, as are women who develop significant gastrointestinal side-effects such as nausea or dyspepsia with oral oestrogens. A few women seem unable to achieve therapeutic plasma levels despite high doses of oral oestrogens probably because of defective oestrogen absorption, and this group will also benefit from the non-oral route. Oral oestrogens are cheaper and this may be a consideration if tight budgetary control is essential.

6.9 What are the principal oral oestrogens?

These were shown in Table. 6.1. Premarin® (Wyeth-Ayerst) and Progynova® (Schering) are the most commonly prescribed preparations in the UK. As discussed in Question 6.4, regardless of the type of oestrogen taken orally the principal plasma product will be oestrone. Consequently, if a patient does not have a satisfactory therapeutic response or develops side-effects with one oral preparation there seems little to be gained in switching to another oral preparation. With a sub-optimal response the dose should be increased, and if oral oestrogens cause significant gastrointestinal side-effects then it makes more sense to alter the route of administration. Harmogen® is useful for administering very low oestrogen doses. A half of one tablet can be particularly valuable as a supplement in the treatment of premenstrual flushes and sweats etc., as discussed in Questions 5.17 and 5.18.

6.10 What are the advantages and disadvantages of the oral route?

These are shown in Table 6.3 and have been discussed in detail in Questions 6.4 and 6.6.

6.11 What is the mechanism of action of the transdermal therapeutic system (TTS)?

Oestrogens are lipid soluble substances which, it is currently believed, cannot penetrate the epidermis of the skin unless they are dissolved in an appropriate transport medium such as ethanol. The oestradiol-TTS patch (Estraderm® : Ciba-Geigy) is a thin, transparent, multilayered unit with an outer impermeable membrane. Oestradiol dissolved in alcohol is contained in high concentrations in the central drug reservoir which is sealed and separated from the epidermis by a permeable rate-controlling membrane. The patch is held in place on the skin by an outer adhesive layer. The alcohol diffuses through the pores of the rate-controlling membrane, across the outer layers of the epidermis along the concentration gradient, and carries the oestradiol with it. Each patch delivers a constant dose of oestradiol for approximately 72 hours. Although less than 10% of the oestradiol within the reservoir is used, most of the alcohol has disappeared by this time and further absorption is reduced. Thus, patches need to be changed every 3–4 days. The rate of drug delivery is determined by the surface area of the patch in contact with the skin. There are currently three sizes available, TTS 25, 50 and 100 which deliver 25, 50 and 100 μg of oestradiol, respectively, into the circulation over a 24-hour period. It is stressed that the dose of oestradiol cannot be increased by changing the patch more frequently.

6.12 What are the advantages and disadvantages of the transdermal therapeutic system?

These are shown in Table 6.3. Most of these points have already been discussed. Skin reactions are quite common with up to 30% of patients experiencing some irritation or erythema at the site of patch application. Although this can be troublesome various strategies exist to reduce this problem and only about 4% of patients actually discontinue this form of treatment for this reason. In our experience, the buttock appears to be the site least prone to skin irritation in most women. Other strategies for overcoming the problems of skin irritation are: (1) rotating the patch site every 24–48 hours (but reapplying the old patch); (2) allowing the patch to stand with the backing strip removed for 10–15 seconds before application to the skin thus allowing any surface alcohol to evaporate (long exposure to the open air is counter-productive as once all the alcohol has evaporated no further absorption of oestradiol can take place), and (3) warning patients that the use of patches in hot, humid climates may increase the risk of skin reactions. Under these circumstances, we advise patients to leave the patch off for the 4–6 hours when on the beach or to switch to oral therapy for the few weeks each year when they are on holiday. The risk of skin reactions may also be increased if the patch is applied to an area of skin covered with talc or perfume.

Transdermal progestogens are currently under development but at present are not licensed for use in the UK.

6.13 What are oestradiol implants?

These are biodegradable crystalline pellets of oestradiol. They are inserted subcutaneously and slowly release oestradiol over many months. Three doses are available, 25 mg, 50 mg and 100 mg. The higher the dose the longer the duration of action.

6.14 What are the advantages and disadvantages of implants?

These are shown in Table 6.3. Implants require a minor surgical procedure for insertion. This is a simple technique that can easily be performed in an outpatient clinic under a local anaesthetic. It is also a technique that can be readily performed by a suitably experienced general practitioner, but the cost of the initial equipment, its maintenance and sterilization may not make it cost-effective if only a few patients in the practice receive this form of therapy. The insertion of implants requires medical skills which ties the patient to periodic follow-up visits. Unlike all other routes of administration, compliance is ensured. However, if a patient develops a significant side-effect then implants are difficult to remove.

Although the stated duration of action is between 4 and 8 months depending upon the dose, this may be an underestimate and there are reports of oestrogenic activity, sufficient to cause endometrial stimulation, continuing for up to 3 years after last insertion. In women with an intact uterus, the progestogen must still be taken every month during this time to prevent endometrial hyperplasia, and this should be continued until withdrawal bleeding has completely ceased. In consequence, progestogens may have to be continued for many, many months if not for up to 2 to 3 years after the decision to stop treatment.

Because many women elect to discontinue therapy because of progestogenic side-effects such as a dislike of the withdrawal bleeding, the 'carry-over' effect can be a disadvantage. But, with proper explanation, it can be overcome. Another disadvantage of implant therapy, tachyphylaxis, is, in our experience, much more difficult to deal with.

6.15 What is tachyphylaxis and how can it be managed?

This is a term used to describe a phenomenon that has been observed principally with implant therapy but which, we suspect, may occur with other routes of administration. Insertion of the first implant is followed by a rapid rise in plasma oestradiol levels and a plateau is reached after some weeks. Patients may begin to experience a recurrence of symptoms as the oestradiol levels fall below this plateau, even though the plasma level is well within the normal premenopausal range. It is not known why this occurs. The return of symptoms leads the patient to encourage the practitioner to insert a further implant. This results in a further rise in plasma levels which are not maintained: as they fall, symptoms return and the process is repeated. This sequence is illustrated, diagrammatically, in Figure 6.3. Eventually, supra-physiological levels of oestradiol may develop and may co-exist in a patient who, paradoxically, still has symptoms of oestrogen deficiency. Some patients, at the same time, experience symptoms of overdosage such as breast tenderness, nausea and bloating. Eventually, the duration of benefit after implantation is minimal, often only a few weeks.

We have found that management of patients with tachyphylaxis is extremely difficult. No agreed strategy exists but we believe that essentially the patient has to go through a withdrawal phase during which the plasma oestradiol levels gradually fall to within the normal, premenopausal range. This can be a long, slow and uncomfortable experience for both patient and practitioner as the woman may experience very distressing symptoms during this time. Supplements of oestradiol, such as transdermal patches, may be used when the symptoms are particularly severe but high doses, $150-200$ μg/day may have to be administered to be beneficial. As far as is known, these will not interfere with the overall process of degradation of the implant. The most important factor in the management of these patients is a careful explanation to the patient of what is happening. An awareness of the potential for this troublesome problem should prevent its development.

Thus, for patients on implants, the temptation to reinsert implants more frequently than every 6 months should be resisted. Monitoring of plasma oestradiol levels, if available, is particularly helpful if symptoms are recurring sooner than expected.

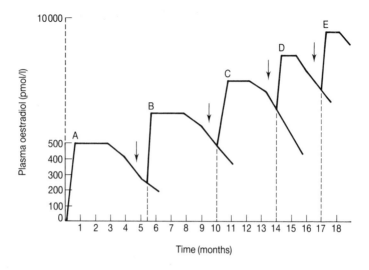

Figure 6.3   Diagrammatic representation of tachyphylaxis. A, B, C, D and E indicate the insertion of new implants. Arrows indicate the recurrence of menopausal symptoms. See text for details. Note ever-decreasing time intervals between implants.

6.16 What are the plasma oestradiol values achieved with implant therapy?

We find this a difficult question to answer because, leaving aside inter-patient variation in absorption and metabolism, the values are likely to depend upon the dose, the frequency of re-implantation and, perhaps, the total duration of administration. Published reports indicate that after insertion of one 50 mg implant plasma levels are maintained above approximately 400 pmol/l for 4 months. In patients receiving 50 mg implants at 6-monthly intervals over a 3-year period, the mean plasma oestradiol value was 625 pmol/l 6 months after insertion of the last implant. We can only speculate as to the values 2–3 months after the last implantation.

We suspect that since our observations on supra-physiological concentrations were reported, practitioners have started to measure plasma oestradiol values more routinely. The majority of our patients receiving 50 mg implants every 5–7 months have plasma oestradiol values between 550 pmol/l and 1100 pmol/l when they request further implantation. Thus, the oestradiol values achieved with implants appear to be considerably higher than those with oral and transdermal therapies (see Fig. 6.1).

6.17 How common is tachyphylaxis and is there a predictive stereotype?

The incidence is not known but most practitioners immediately recognize the phenomenon when described.

It has been suggested that women who have undergone premature, surgical menopause (who are more likely to receive implants) and those with a history of psychiatric disorder are more likely to develop tachyphylaxis. Confirmatory data are awaited.

6.18 Are the higher plasma oestradiol values that some patients attain with implants likely to be beneficial or harmful?

This is not known. If the effects of oestradiol on bone, arterial disease and breast cancer risk are dose-related, then implants will exert greater benefits on bone and arterial disease risk but will increase the risk of breast cancer. It is doubtful whether implants will dramatically increase oestrogen benefits on arterial disease risk because these do not appear dose-related (see Question 4.41).

6.19 What are testosterone implants and when should they be used?

Testosterone is an androgen and is produced by the ovary. Castration removes this endogenous source. The precise role of testosterone in women is unclear and the literature is contradictory. However, in our experience it appears to have a beneficial effect on libido and energy levels in some women. Testosterone is usually administered in implant form. We use testosterone implants following castration, and in those women in whom there is a refractory loss of libido or loss of energy despite an otherwise good therapeutic response to oestrogens. Testosterone implants have the potential to cause virilising side-effects such as hirsutism and deepening of the voice. We have never seen the latter: hirsutism occurs rarely and if further testosterone implants are withheld it resolves spontaneously. The dose we use is 50/100 mg implanted every 6–8 months — to minimize the risk of side-effects we prefer the lower dose.

6.20 Does the addition of the testosterone influence the effects of oestrogen on bone response or arterial disease risk?

This is not known.

6.21 What is recommended for the treatment of localized atrophic changes of the urogenital tract?

Many women presenting solely with these problems will be some years after menopause. The prospect of the return of regular vaginal bleeding may be a deterrent in this age group. Therefore, many will prefer the use of vaginal oestrogen preparations.

In the past, it was believed that vaginal creams acted only locally. However, more recent studies have shown that a significant but variable amount of oestrogen is absorbed into the systemic circulation via the vaginal epithelium. The use of vaginal oestrogens at high dose and long term increases the risk of endometrial cancer. Thus, to achieve only local effects within the lower urogenital tract, vaginal oestrogens must be administered at low dose. An increase in dose, either undertaken deliberately by the patient or by using the vaginal oestrogen as a lubricant, may result in significant systemic absorption and effects upon distant but dependent end-organs.

6.22 What oestrogens are available for vaginal administration?

These are shown in Table 6.1. The preparations are based on conjugated equine oestrogens (as per the oral formulation), oestradiol or oestriol. All three are classified as natural oestrogens. Oestriol is often described as a 'weak' oestrogen but such a description is subject to misinterpretation. Unlike the other natural oestrogens, oestriol is not strongly bound in plasma to albumin or SHBG and circulates largely in an unbound form. The majority of a loading dose of oestriol is excreted within 8 hours. Thus, once daily administration of a low dose imparts but a small oestrogenic stimulus. However, when administered in divided daily doses and at high dose, oestriol exerts identical intracellular responses to oestradiol in mammalian species, and can cause endometrial hyperplasia in postmenopausal women. For reasons not fully understood, high dose oestriol therapy does not appear to protect against postmenopausal bone loss. Thus, with once daily administration at low dose oestriol appears to exert an effect upon the lower urogenital tract but has little systemic effect.

6.23 How are vaginal oestrogens best prescribed?

The rate of systemic absorption from the vagina may increase as the epithelium becomes more oestrogenized, presumably because of increased vascularity. Thus, when starting treatment with vaginal oestrogens, the preparation (cream/tablet) should be inserted 4−5 times weekly for the first few weeks and then reduced to twice-weekly insertion. The precise dosage at which vaginal oestrogens start to have a significant systemic effect (e.g. endometrial stimulation) is not known. We would regard the manufacturers' recommended dose of conjugated equine oestrogens as likely to cause systemic effects if administered every day. We would suggest that they be administered twice weekly. A once-daily dose of oestriol does not appear to affect the endometrium. If the patient or practitioner has concerns about endometrial stimulation then progestogen addition can be considered.

A progestogen challenge test performed after 3 months may be helpful. This involves administering an oral progestogen for 10−12 consecutive days; the recommended daily progestogen doses are discussed in Question 6.35. If withdrawal bleeding occurs following progestogen withdrawal, then endometrial stimulation is occurring and monthly progestogen addition would seem advisable. If no bleeding occurs then the progestogen challenge test can be repeated after an interval of some months.

It is important to advise women not to use vaginal oestrogen creams as a lubricant as significant absorption by the partner has been reported.

6.24 Can vaginal oestrogens be used as lubricants?

They can but the higher dose may result in systemic effects. Furthermore, significant absorption of the oestrogen through the penile skin and into the systemic circulation of the partner has been reported. Rarely, gynaecomastia may result.

6.25 Can vaginal oestrogens be given with other oestrogen treatments?

Yes. In many women systemic treatment (pills, patches or implants), by itself, will be sufficient to improve their vaginal dryness and dyspareunia. However, in some women the lower urogenital tract symptoms are a refractory problem despite standard doses of systemic HRT (see Question 6.27). Under these circumstances, the addition of a vaginal oestrogen preparation can be helpful.

6.26 What are the advantages and disadvantages of the vaginal route?

The use of the vaginal route to obtain systemic benefits (relief of flushes/sweats etc.) has largely been superseded by other routes of administration. We have a few patients who cannot take oral oestrogens because of gastrointestinal side-effects, cannot tolerate transdermal therapy because of skin reactions and will not consider implants. For them, vaginal oestrogens are a suitable alternative but administration has to be on a daily basis. Because of the low oestrogen stimulus achieved with once-daily oestriol, we tend to prescribe vaginal conjugated equine oestrogens 2–4 gm each night. The potential disadvantage to the partner of high dose vaginal oestrogen creams has already been mentioned. With such doses, oral progestogens need to be added in non-hysterectomized women.

While twice-weekly administration of conjugated equine oestrogens or daily administration of oestriol tablets or creams will relieve lower urogenital tract symptoms and may not cause withdrawal bleeding, the oestrogenic stimulus is too low for bone conservation and it is most unlikely that it will achieve the arterial benefits seen with other routes of administration.

6.27 What dose of oral, transdermal and subcutaneous (implant) oestrogens should be prescribed?

This depends entirely upon the indication for treatment. Appropriate oestrogen doses for the various indications are shown in Table 6.4. For most women, the 'standard' dose (middle column) will be sufficient. Not only will this relieve troublesome symptoms but it will also prevent significant bone loss. Thus, it represents the ideal starting dose. However, women with severe symptoms may require a higher dose (right-hand column), and in our experience this applies particularly to women who have undergone a premature, surgical menopause. Even the highest doses with the oral and transdermal routes do not result in plasma oestradiol values above those seen in the normal peri-ovulatory phase of the menstrual cycle (Figure 6.1), and thus the practitioner need not have undue concerns about increasing above the standard dose if the situation demands it. It appears that even on the 'standard' oral and transdermal HRT doses a few women will not conserve bone (see Question 4.25). Therefore, if this is the principal indication for HRT then due consideration should be given to serial bone density measurements. Alternatively, a higher dose may be prescribed, particularly if the therapeutic response is sub-optimal.

Rarely, the standard doses cause symptoms of oestrogen excess such as severe, continuing breast tenderness, nipple sensitivity, leg cramps and weight gain. These problems are discussed further in Question 7.2. These side-effects are more likely to be seen in women in the late climacteric who are still menstruating, albeit erratically. They arise when surges of spontaneous ovarian activity occur, and the combination of endogenous and

Table 6.4 Daily dosages of various oestrogen preparations for use in postmenopausal women according to symptom relief and bone conservation

	Symptom relief			Bone conservation
	Vaginal dryness	Mild/moderate vasomotor symptoms ('standard' dose)	Severe vasomotor symptoms	Minimum bone conserving dose (in majority of women)
Premarin®	0.625 mg cream twice weekly	0.625 mg	1.25 mg	0.625 mg
Progynova®	1 mg	1−2 mg	2−4mg	2 mg
Estraderm®	25 µg	50 µg	100 µg	50 µg
Oestradiol implant	25 mg	25−50 mg	50−100 mg	50 mg

spontaneous ovarian activity occur, and the combination of endogenous and exogenous oestrogen results in excess. These surges of ovarian activity tend to be intermittent and may last from a few days to some weeks. In most women, the symptoms of oestrogen excess resolve spontaneously as ovarian function declines. However, if the symptoms persist then dosage reduction is indicated.

For women who have very minor symptoms or in whom vaginal dryness is the only problem, the lower doses (left-hand column) may be used. However, it must be pointed out that these doses have not been shown to be bone sparing or to protect against arterial disease risk.

6.28 Should the same doses be prescribed to women starting HRT who are many years postmenopausal?

Our current understanding is that the dosage requirements do not change with time after menopause. Thus, in a 70-year-old woman starting HRT to reduce the risk of later osteoporotic fracture the maintenance dose will be the same as in an early postmenopausal woman. However, in the older woman starting HRT after several years of oestrogen deficiency, it is advisable to start with a low dose for 6−12 weeks and then to increase to the standard dose. In women many years after menopause, standard doses if used to initiate therapy may cause troublesome side-effects, particularly breast tenderness, nipple sensitivity and leg cramps. The older woman should be advised that these side-effects may even occur with the lower oestrogen doses but that they do not represent breast cancer or thrombotic disease.

6.29 What is the relationship between the oestrogen dose and the likelihood of withdrawal bleeding being established?

Little information is available to address this question. It is stressed that withdrawal bleeding will only occur if the oestrogenic stimulus is sufficient to cause endometrial stimulation, and if the progestogen is administered at adequate daily dose and for sufficient duration (see Question 6.35). Assuming that the latter criteria are fulfilled, it is to be expected that the percentage of women experiencing withdrawal bleeding will rise as the oestrogen dose is increased. In our experience, almost all patients receiving oestradiol implants experience withdrawal bleeding, and this most probably reflects the more than adequate plasma oestradiol levels achieved with this form of therapy. With conjugated equine oestrogens 0.625 mg/day (or an equivalent such as transdermal oestradiol, 50 μg/day), approximately 85% of women experience withdrawal bleeding: the remainder do not. The absence of bleeding is not a cause for concern and endometrial biopsy is not indicated because of amenorrhoea. The lack of bleeding in this minority most probably reflects the wide inter-patient variation in plasma oestradiol values achieved with all therapies (see Question 6.5).

Few data are available with lower doses administered systemically, such as transdermal oestradiol 25 μg/day. In our experience, approximately 50% of patients experience withdrawal bleeding with this dose when a progestogen is added.

6.30 Should oestrogens be prescribed cyclically or continuously?

The principal aim of HRT is to replace levels of oestrogen which are deficient after the menopause. Premenopausally, the ovary produces oestrogen continuously although the levels fluctuate throughout the ovarian cycle (see Fig. 6.1). There seems to be no advantage in re-creating the peri-ovulatory peak seen premenopausally and the aim with HRT is to achieve a consistent, therapeutic plasma level of oestrogen.

Consequently, with HRT, we believe that the oestrogen should be prescribed continuously. We see no advantage in prescribing the oestrogen cyclically, i.e. for 3 weeks out of 4. Stopping treatment for 7 days each cycle only results in the return of troublesome symptoms in a number of patients. It confers no protection to the endometrium, nor is there any evidence that it has a beneficial effect on the breast. Thus, with systemic therapy, we believe that the oestrogen should be prescribed continuously for 365 days a year.

PROGESTOGENS

6.31 What types of progestogens are available?

If, for classification purposes, we apply the same criteria to progestogens as for oestrogens then there is only one 'natural' preparation which is progesterone. All other progestogens are 'synthetic' in that they are structurally dissimilar to substances produced by the ovary.

The synthetic progestogens have been classified in a variety of ways. The simplest classification subdivides them into two major groups: (1) those that are structurally related to progesterone, e.g. medroxyprogesterone acetate and dydrogesterone, and (2) those structurally related to testosterone, e.g. norethisterone and norgestrel. The 'new' generation of progestogens, desogestrel, norgestimate and gestodene are all derivates of norgestrel. By manipulation of the parent molecule, it is claimed that the progestogenic potency of these substances is enhanced relative to their androgenic activity.

6.32 Why isn't natural progesterone used in HRT?

Because progesterone is one of the precursors of many other types of steroids (apart from sex hormones), numerous enzyme systems exist which rapidly metabolize this hormone. Many of these are to be found within the liver and therefore oral administration results in a relatively small increase in plasma progesterone concentrations, with similar and much larger increases in the circulating concentrations of the principal metabolites. Because of this rapid metabolism, oral progesterone needs to be given in divided daily doses if an adequate endometrial effect is to be achieved in all women. This can be effected with 200 mg oral progesterone administered at night with a further 100 mg given in the morning. At these doses, drowsiness is a common complaint (hence the use of 200 mg oral progesterone at night), and the sedative effects of high doses of progesterone have been recognized for many years. There is a wide inter-patient variation in absorption and metabolism of oral progesterone, and peak values for progesterone can vary as much as three-fold between individuals.

The non-oral route may permit therapeutic plasma concentrations, maintained over 24 hours, with once-daily administration. Natural progesterone is well absorbed both vaginally and rectally, and suppositories are available in doses of 200 mg and 400 mg. However, there are sparse data on the endometrial effects of these doses when so administered, and in our experience these routes of administration are not well tolerated by British women.

6.33 How can the potency of the different synthetic progestogens be assessed?

Various assay systems exist using the response of certain tissues of lower mammals. However, the validity of extrapolating these data to the human situation is questionable because progestogens exert dissimilar effects in different animal species (e.g. they cause endometrial proliferation in some).

There is no ideal classification of progestogen potency in postmenopausal women. Because progestogens are added to reduce the risk of endometrial hyperstimulation, we think it makes most sense to determine their relative potencies with respect to the endometrial response. Because some progestogens are rapidly metabolized when given orally, relative potencies determined from oral administration may not apply when a non-oral route of administration is utilized.

6.34 Why are progestogens added to oestrogen in HRT?

Progestogens are added to oestrogens to protect the endometrium. Prospective, histological studies have reported an 18–32% incidence of endometrial hyperplasia with oral oestrogen therapy alone; up to one third were of the more sinister atypical variety which carries a higher risk of subsequent malignant change. The incidence of hyperplasia is significantly reduced by adding a progestogen, and it is stressed that the protective effects are both dose and duration dependent. With a relatively high dose of norethisterone, 5 mg/day, one research group in the UK reported that the incidence of hyperplasia in women receiving oestradiol implants was reduced from 9% with 5 days of norethisterone added each month, to 3% with 10 days and to zero with 13 days. Another UK group which prescribed oral oestrogens reported similar data, the incidence of hyperplasia being 3–4% with 7 days, 2% with 10 days and zero with 12 days when the progestogen dose was kept high. However, when the latter group reduced the progestogen dose, hyperplasia was observed even in patients adding progestogen for 12 days each calendar month/cycle. Thus, an adequate daily dose prescribed for an inadequate duration, or an adequate duration but inadequate daily dose may both result in hyperplasia.

As compared to unopposed, cyclical oestrogen therapy, the incidence of endometrial carcinoma is significantly reduced when combined oestrogen/progestogen regimens are used. It is not clear whether combination therapies reduce the risk to below that seen in an untreated population (see Question 8.33).

6.35 What are the optimal doses of progestogens required with oral and transdermal oestrogens, and how can they be determined?

Progestogenic effects upon the endometrium have been assessed both histologically and biochemically.

Histological evaluation has included conventional light microscopy of endometrial tissue obtained using either a Vabra suction curette or at conventional dilatation and curettage under general anaesthesia. In addition, transmission electron microscopy has been used to determine the presence of certain intracellular, ultra-structural features which are induced by progesterone after ovulation in premenopausal women.

Progestogens appear to exert their protective effects through two mechanisms. Firstly they oppose oestrogenic stimulation and thereby reduce the mitotic or proliferative effects of oestrogen. Thus, the anti-mitotic or anti-proliferative effects of progestogens can be quantified through determining the suppression of deoxyribonucleic acid (DNA) synthesis and nuclear oestradiol receptor levels. Secondly, by causing secretory transformation, progestogens induce certain enzymes which are not only involved in the metabolism of oestradiol but which also are partially responsible for autolysis following progestogen withdrawal. Autolysis leads to cell death and, in conjunction with other mechanisms, menstruation ensues. Thus, potentially neoplastic cells are shed. It is not known whether the anti-mitotic or secretory effects of progestogens are more important in affording protection against endometrial carcinoma, or whether they are equally important.

The histological and biochemical data upon the effects of progestogens on the endometrium have been in broad agreement. The minimum effective daily doses of various orally administered progestogens when added for 10–12 days each calendar month to oral and transdermal oestrogens are shown in Table 6.5.

6.36 Are these doses satisfactory for all patients on oral and transdermal oestrogens?

No. Both biochemically and histologically there is a variation in response to any dose of any progestogen. This is why some of the doses are given as ranges. The reasons for the inter-patient variation in response are unclear but possible explanations include inter-patient variation in absorption and metabolism of the administered steroid, and/or variations in endometrial sensitivity.

This wide inter-patient variation in response to progestogen may imply that routine endometrial biopsy is required in all patients receiving HRT.

Table 6.5 Recommended daily dose ranges of various progestogens for use with oral/transdermal oestrogens

Chemical name	Dose	Brand name and dose
Norethisterone	0.7/1.05 mg	(Micronor®/Noriday® 2−3 tablets)
	to 2.5 mg	(one half of a 5 mg tablet)
L-Norgestrel	150 μg	(Neogest® 2 tablets)
Dydrogesterone	10−20 mg	(Duphaston® 1−2 tablets)
Medroxyprogesterone acetate	10 mg	(Provera® 2 tablets)

However, observation of the withdrawal bleeding pattern of women on combined oral oestrogen/progestogen preparations has shown a useful correlation between the day of onset of bleeding and the histological type of endometrium. Similar data exist for transdermal oestrogen/oral progestogen combinations (see Question 9.30 and Fig. 9.3). Thus, the pattern of onset of bleeding can be used to predict the endometrial status with these routes of oestrogen administration.

6.37 Are these doses of progestogens effective in patients receiving oestradiol implants?

We have not performed similar dose-ranging studies of various progestogens in patients receiving oestradiol implants. Because of the higher plasma oestradiol values that some patients achieve with implant therapy, we would urge caution in extrapolating the progestogen doses shown in Table 6.5 to patients receiving oestradiol implants. Data are available that higher daily doses of norethisterone, 5 mg/day, are protective. However, the higher the progestogen dose the greater the likelihood of progestogen-induced symptomatic and psychological side-effects. Our practice is to prescribe the lowest dose of an oral progestogen which results in withdrawal bleeding which reliably starts on the 11th−12th day of progestogen addition (if the progestogen is given for 12 days), or thereafter (usually within 24−72 hours of stopping the progestogen). In patients who start to bleed on the seventh or eighth day of progestogen addition, irrespective of the preparation, we increase the dose until the withdrawal bleeding starts at the appropriate time as stated above. In our practice, we usually initiate therapy with norethisterone 2.5 mg/day or with dydrogesterone 20 mg/day for 12 days each calendar month, and review the patient for adjustment of the progestogen dosage after 4−6 months. If the withdrawal bleeding is starting many days after the progestogen has been withdrawn (around 7−10 days after discontinuation), then a dosage reduction can be tried.

6.38 What routes of administration are available for progestogens?

The most commonly employed route of administration is the oral route. While natural progesterone can be administered either vaginally or rectally, there are scant data on the doses required for endometrial protection.

Currently, the transdermal route of administration for progestogens is receiving considerable attention. Preliminary data indicate that this is a safe and effective method of administering progestogens. As compared to the oral route, the dose of certain progestogens may be reduced by approximately 75% with transdermal administration yet endometrial effects are still observed. Because of the lower dose, the symptomatic and psychological side-effects associated with progestogen use appear to be minimized. It is anticipated that transdermal progestogens will become available in the UK in the near future.

Depo-progestogens are available but there are no data upon their effects when combined with oestrogen. We would predict a high incidence of irregular bleeding as this strategy is a form of continuous/combined, oestrogen/progestogen therapy (see Question 9.30).

COMBINED OESTROGEN/PROGESTOGEN PREPARATIONS

Progestogens may be added sequentially to the oestrogen for durations ranging from 7–12 days each cycle. For reasons discussed elsewhere (see Question 6.34), we prefer a minimum of 12 days of progestogen addition. Such combined/sequential oestrogen/progestogen therapy usually results in withdrawal bleeding. To try to induce amenorrhoea, research has been undertaken on continuous/combined oestrogen/progestogen regimens in which a small dose of progestogen is added to the oestrogen, every day. Because of the problems with chronic, irregular bleeding and because of the lack of long-term safety data we do not recommend the use of continuous/combined therapies in general practice at this time (see also Question 9.30).

6.39 How should I prescribe combined/sequential oestrogen/progestogen therapy?

Calendar packs in which the oestrogen and progestogen are combined are commercially available and are considered further below. An alternative approach is to prescribe oestrogen and progestogen separately. This does not involve the patient in extra expense because combination packs carry a double prescription charge. Separate prescription is the method which we have used extensively for many years because it allows much greater flexibility in timing of administration and adjustment of dosage of the progestogen. The method involves the use of oral, transdermal, subcutaneous or vaginal oestrogens administered continuously, i.e. for 365 days per year. The progestogen is added at appropriate dose (see Table 6.5 and Question 6.37) for the first 12 days of each *calendar month*, i.e. the course of progestogen is commenced on the 1st January, 1st February, 1st March, etc. We have found that this method is popular and compliance is rarely a problem.

6.40 What are the advantages of prescribing the oestrogen and progestogen separately?

Patients find the schedule easy to follow and can mark off in their diary or wall calendar when to take the progestogen. The withdrawal bleeding will start around the same time each month (usually between the 11th and the 14th of the month), and will last for approximately 4–6 days. If in a certain month the bleeding will occur at a socially undesirable time (holiday, weekend social event), then the patient can advance or retard the timing of progestogen addition by up to 7–10 days so as to avoid bleeding at the undesired time. Or, alternatively, can miss out the progestogen in that month. The nursing staff know that if a compliant patient on such a regimen phones later in the month (after day 20) complaining of current bleeding then further investigation is required (see Question 9.40). As discussed in Questions 6.35 and 6.37, patients whose withdrawal bleeding starts early during the phase of progestogen addition can have the dose increased; dosage reductions may also be indicated if the withdrawal bleeding does not start until 7–10 days after the progestogen has been withdrawn.

For reasons not understood but discussed in greater detail in Question 7.10, some patients may experience significant side-effects with a certain progestogen but these may be minimised or abolished by changing to another preparation. Thus, intolerance to norethisterone or norgestrel may be overcome by changing to medroxyprogesterone acetate or dydrogesterone, and vice versa. This can easily be effected by prescribing the oestrogen and progestogen separately.

Lastly, separate prescription can be of value in the perimenopausal woman with a menstrual cycle which is regular but which is not of 28 days' duration. If oestrogen-deficiency symptoms occur only premenstrually, then oestrogen supplementation can be adopted in the premenstrual phase (see Questions 5.16 and 5.18). However, if the symptoms occur throughout the cycle then the oestrogen needs to be given continuously. The progestogen is prescribed so that the last tablet is taken the day before the first day of the next, expected period. Thus, with a cycle length of 24 days the progestogen is added from day 12 (counting the first day of normal menstrual bleeding as day 1) through to day 23; with a cycle length of 40 days, the progestogen is added from day 28 through to day 39. This overcomes the problem of a fixed, 28-day treatment cycle which is used in all combination packs and which, when given to perimenopausal women with a different length of cycle, tends to cause breakthrough bleeding (see Question 5.16).

6.41 What are the disadvantages of prescribing the oestrogen and progestogen separately?

Compliance. It is all too easy for the patient to avoid taking the progestogen. The need for progestogen addition in non-hysterectomized women must be clearly understood.

6.42 What combined preparations or 'packs' are available?

At present, four combined preparations are available; all use natural oestrogens with a synthetic progestogen (Table 6.6). Three of these preparations contain an oral oestrogen and an oral progestogen, and the fourth is a combination of transdermal oestradiol patches together with an oral progestogen.

6.43 What are the advantages of combination packs?

All are designed to be 'user-friendly' and to encourage compliance. Certain criticisms can be made of various combinations. We favour preparations which deliver the oestrogen continuously, throughout the cycle (see Question 6.30). Cyclo-Progynova® (Schering: oestradiol valerate/ norgestrel) has a 7-day oestrogen-free week each month, and the daily dose of the progestogen is in excess of that required for endometrial protection. We suspect that this preparation may be reformulated in the near future. Trisequens® (Novo: oestradiol/oestriol/norethisterone) contains two oestrogens, oestradiol and oestriol. We understand that the latter was added because of a belief that it would impede the action of oestradiol on vulnerable end-organs (such as the endometrium) and reduce the risk of hyperstimulation. Recently, this has been shown to be a fallacy. While the norethisterone is given at low dose, 1 mg/day, it is only added for 10 days. Two research groups have reported that 10 days of progestogen addition carried a 2% risk of hyperplasia.

Table 6.6 HRT combination packs currently available

Oestrogen duration	Progestogen duration	Proprietary name
Conjugated equine oestrogens 0.625 mg/28 days	Norgestrel 150 μg/12 days	Prempak-C® 0.625
Conjugated equine oestrogens 1.25 mg/28 days	Norgestrel 150 μg/12 days	Prempak-C® 1.25
Oestradiol + oestriol (various doses)/28 days	Norethisterone 1 mg/10 days	Trisequens®
Oestradiol valerate 2 mg/21 days	Norgestrel 500 μg/10 days	Cyclo-Progynova® 2 mg
Oestradiol valerate 1 mg/21 days	Norgestrel 500 μg/10 days	Cyclo-Progynova® 1 mg
Transdermal oestradiol 50 μg/28 days	Norethisterone 1 mg/12 days	Estrapak®

Cyclo-Progynova ® and Trisequens ® possess one advantage over Prempak-C® (Wyeth: conjugated equine oestrogen/norgestrel) and Estrapak® (Ciba: transdermal oestradiol/norethisterone). In the former two preparations, the progestogen is supplied in the same tablet as the oestrogen and it is impossible for the patient to be non-compliant with the progestogen.

6.44 What are the disadvantages of combination packs?

While these packs have undoubted advantages in terms of encouraging compliance, it is not easy to adjust the timing of progestogen administration nor to tailor the dose to suit an individual patient. With certain preparations, i.e. Prempak-C® and Estrapak®, the progestogen is provided in a separate tablet and therefore there is a potential for non-compliance despite the fact that the calendar pack is intended to encourage compliance.

All the combination packs contain either norethisterone or norgestrel, and both are derivatives of testosterone. Thus, if a patient develops side-effects due likely to the androgenic potency of the progestogen (greasy skin, acne), changing therapy to another combination may not overcome the problem. Prescribing the oestrogen separately together with a progesterone derivative, such as medroxyprogesterone acetate or dydrogesterone, makes much more sense. Similarly, if the progestogen in Prempak-C® is poorly tolerated and causes significant side-effects then changing to Cyclo-Progynova® is unlikely to be of benefit: both contain the same progestogen.

Combination packs containing medroxyprogesterone acetate or dydrogesterone are not available.

6.45 What are the relative costs?

The approximate costs of a month's supply of oestrogen-alone, progestogen-alone and the combination preparations are given in Table 6.7.

RECOMMENDED DOSES

6.46 What is the 'standard' starting dose of HRT?

For the oestrogen, this was discussed in Question 6.27 and illustrated in Table 6.4; in a non-hysterectomized woman, the daily dose of the available progestogens was shown in Table 6.5.

With combination therapies, the standard starting dose is Prempak-C® 0.625 mg, Cyclo-Progynova® 2 mg or Estrapak 50®. In patients with severe symptoms Prempak-C 1.25 mg is available. All these preparations together with Trisequens® should, on current evidence, afford skeletal protection against osteoporosis in the majority of women. However, it is unlikely that Cyclo-Progynova® 1 mg will be as effective as a bone conserver because of the lower oestrogen dose.

The importance of starting therapy with a lower oestrogen dose in the older woman was referred to in Question 6.28. This may be achieved with transdermal oestradiol, 25 μg/day, oestradiol valerate, 1 mg/day, conjugated equine oestrogens, half of an 0.625 mg tablet a day or 0.625 mg on alternate days, or piperazine oestrone sulphate, 0.75 mg/day. The dose can be increased to a standard regimen, if indicated, after the initial 6–12-week adjustment period has passed, and in the absence of significant oestrogen-dependent side-effects.

6.47 What is the most appropriate route of administration as 'first-line' therapy?

We favour either the oral or transdermal route as first-line therapy in all patients, except those who have undergone castration at a young age. There are obvious advantages with these routes in that dosage adjustment is facilitated, and perhaps more importantly therapy can easily be discontinued if necessary. In the young castrate, we favour testosterone implants with either oestradiol implants inserted concurrently or, in those patients requesting re-implantation at ever-decreasing intervals, testosterone implants with transdermal oestradiol, 100 μg/day.

We stress that medical opinion on the issue of first-line therapy is divided and that some authorities would recommend implants from the beginning.

Table 6.7 Approximate monthly costs of various hormone preparations in current usage for HRT (source: MIMS)

Brand name	Dose	£
Premarin®	0.625 mg	1.38
	1.25 mg	2.25
Progynova®	1 mg	2.64
	2 mg	2.64
Estraderm®	25 μg	6.75
	50 μg	7.45
	100 μg	8.20
Micronor®⎫ Noriday® ⎬	0.7 mg × 12 days	0.54
Neogest®	0.15 mg × 12 days	0.54
Duphaston®	10 mg × 12 days	2.01
	20 mg × 12 days	4.02
Provera®	10 mg × 12 days	3.01
Cyclogest®	200 mg × 12 days	4.32
	400 mg × 12 days	6.27
Prempak-C®	0.625 mg	3.98
	1.25 mg	3.98
Cyclo-Progynova®	1 mg	3.50
	2 mg	3.50
Trisequens®	2 mg	3.74
Estrapak®	50 μg	8.45

6.48 Which patients are likely to derive most benefit from implants?

Those who recommend implants as first-line therapy would, we suspect, answer that all patients are likely to derive most benefit from implants.

We believe that it is probably best to reserve the subcutaneous route of administration for those women who cannot absorb or tolerate oestrogens given via the oral or transdermal routes. Also, women who have undergone hysterectomy are an obvious choice for implant therapy. They do not need progestogens, and with implant therapy can forget about HRT until the next implant is due.

Oestradiol implants may be particularly useful in patients were there is a predominance of psycho-sexual symptoms since testosterone implants, discussed in Question 6.19, can be given concurrently.

7. Side-effects of HRT

Oestrogens and progestogens affect many tissues and their metabolic consequences and long-term influence on vulnerable end-organs, such as the breast and endometrium, are discussed elsewhere. This chapter discusses the physical and psychological changes which result from administration of oestrogens and progestogens, with particular emphasis on those that are undesirable and which arise during the first few months of treatment. Some of the side-effects are common to both oestrogens and progestogens but others are not. Therefore, the two steroids will be discussed separately.

OESTROGENS

7.1 Are peri- and postmenopausal women placebo-responsive?

Yes. Numerous placebo-controlled studies have reported that certain physical and psychological characteristics are influenced as much by placebo as by oestrogen therapy. Certain data from one such study are reproduced in Figure 7.1. They were derived from a prospective, randomized, double-blind placebo-controlled, cross-over study of 61 peri- and postmenopausal women with moderate menopausal symptoms (mainly vasomotor disturbances) who completed a 12-month trial. One half of the patients received conjugated equine oestrogens, 1.25 mg/day, cyclically (for 3 weeks out of 4) for 6 months, followed by an identical placebo which was also given for 6 months; the other half was studied over an identical time but took the placebo first and then the conjugated equine oestrogens. Graphic rating scale assessments (visual analogue) were performed pre-treatment and at 2-monthly intervals during each 6-month treatment course. The mean values over each 6-month course of treatment are presented. Graphic rating scales consist of a 10-cm line with the two ends of the line representing the extremes (very good, very bad; always, never). The data shown here represent the mean change observed during therapy

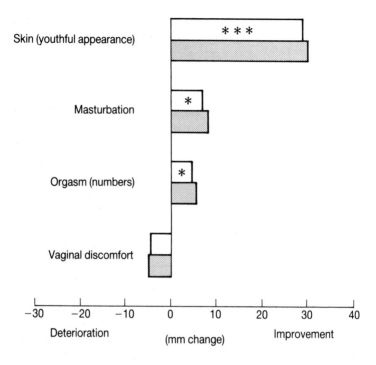

Figure 7.1 Differences in mean graphic rating scale scores as compared to pre-treatment during therapy with conjugated equine oestrogens (▨)or placebo (☐). P values represent significant differences between pre-treatment and treatment scores. ***p < 0.001 *p < 0.05. (From Campbell S, Whitehead M I 1977 In: Greenblatt R B and Studd J W W (eds) Clinics in obstetrics and gynaecology. W B Saunders London and Philadelphia 4 (1): pp 31−47. Reproduced with permission.)

with conjugated equine oestrogens or placebo, irrespective of whether given as the first or second course of treatment, as compared to pre-treatment. The latter is represented by the vertical line.

Conjugated equine oestrogens and placebo caused similar and statistically significant improvements in 'youthful skin appearance', frequency of masturbation and number of orgasms. Similar but non-significant changes were observed for both treatments for vaginal discomfort. The mechanism whereby placebo can exert such significant effects is unknown. It has been suggested that patients experience a general psychological uplift in going to a doctor and receiving sympathy for menopausal ailments. Expectations, also, are clearly important and are discussed further below. The significant placebo effect on 'youthful skin appearance' illustrated here is more understandable in view of beauty parlour publicity, and helps explain the continuing success of such institutions.

Because of this type of placebo response, uncontrolled (i.e. no placebo) studies are of limited value in determining the precise benefits of and side-effects due to exogenous oestrogen administration.

7.2 What physical and psychological side-effects are common after starting oestrogens?

Further data from the study referred to in Question 7.1 are shown in Tables 7.1 and 7.2. Seven symptoms considered to be side-effects of oestrogen treatment were reported by five or more patients. Table 7.1 shows the number of patients reporting each side-effect during therapy with conjugated equine oestrogens or placebo, and Table 7.2 shows the number of patients reporting each side-effect during the first and second courses of treatment (irrespective of the order of administering conjugated equine oestrogens and placebo).

Table 7.1 shows that every symptom was reported more frequently with conjugated equine oestrogens as compared with placebo but, with the exception of leg cramps, the frequency of symptom reporting was low and the differences between active and placebo treatments were small. For example, only 13% of patients reported breast tenderness with conjugated equine oestrogens as compared to 10% with placebo; fluid retention was reported by 8% with oestrogen therapy and by 3% during placebo. The recurrence of a physiological vaginal discharge due to oestrogens was expected, and it is surprising that this was reported by only 8% of women (none with placebo).

Sixteen patients reported leg cramps, 13 during therapy with conjugated equine oestrogens. Although conjugated equine oestrogens are a 'natural' oestrogen, because of the known association between synthetic oestrogens and deep vein thrombosis, [125] I-labelled fibrinogen testing was performed on all 61 patients on two occasions, i.e. before the commencement of the study and at the end of each 6-month treatment period. [125] I-labelled fibrinogen tests were also performed on some patients actually during an episode of leg cramping; no patient was found to have isotopic evidence of venous thrombosis of the legs on any occasion.

The expectation of side-effects upon commencement of oestrogen therapy is illustrated in Table 7.2. All symptoms were reported by more patients during the first course of treatment than during the second whether this was conjugated equine oestrogens or placebo.

From the data shown in Tables 7.1 and 7.2 the authors concluded that the incidence and nature of side-effects was minor. A higher incidence was observed with conjugated equine oestrogens but the difference, as compared

Table 7.1 Side-effects of therapy depending on whether the patient was ingesting equine oestrogens or placebo.

Symptom	Number of patients reporting symptom during Premarin therapy	Number of patients reporting symptom during placebo therapy
Leg cramps [a]	13 (21%)	3 (5%)
Breast tenderness [a]	8 (13%)	6 (10%)
Limb pains	5 (8%)	2 (3%)
Fluid retention	5 (8%)	2 (3%)
Eye irritation [b]	5 (8%)	2 (3%)
Nausea	4 (7%)	2 (3%)
Vaginal discharge	5 (8%)	0 (–)

[a] Two patients reported leg cramps and breast tenderness during both Premarin therapy and placebo therapy.

[b] One patient reported eye irritation during both Premarin therapy and placebo therapy. Premarin = conjugated equine oestrogens.

(From Campbell S, Whitehead M I 1977 In: Greenblatt R B, Studd J W W (eds) Clinics in obstetrics and gynaecology. W B Saunders, London and Philadelphia 4 (1): pp 31–47. Reproduced by permission.)

Table 7.2 Side-effects of therapy reported during the first and second courses of treatment

Symptom	Number of patients reporting symptom during first course of treatment	Number of patients reporting symptom during the second course of treatment
Leg cramps [a]	10 (16%)	6 (10%)
Breast tenderness [a]	10 (16%)	4 (7%)
Limb pains	4 (7%)	3 (5%)
Fluid retention	5 (8%)	2 (3%)
Eye irritation [b]	5 (8%)	2 (3%)
Nausea	4 (7%)	2 (3%)
Vaginal discharge	4 (7%)	1 (2%)

[a] Two patients reported leg cramps and breast tenderness during both the first and second courses of treatment.

[b] One patient reported eye irritation during both the first and second courses of treatment.

(From Campbell S, Whitehead M I 1977 In: Greenblatt R B, Studd J W W (eds) Clinics in obstetrics and gynaecology. W B Saunders, London and Philadelphia 4 (1): pp 31–47. Reproduced with permission.)

to placebo, was small and was most marked for leg cramps. The mechanism whereby oestrogens cause leg cramps is not known but it does not appear to be related to venous thrombosis.

7.3 Do oestrogens cause weight gain?

In the placebo-controlled studies referred to above, weight was assessed pre-treatment and every 2 months during the 12-month study period. The changes in mean values are shown in Figure 7.2; the vertical scale indicates a weight change of ± 1 kg (2 lbs). After the first 2 months of therapy, mean weight had increased in the group taking conjugated equine oestrogens by 0.5 kg (approximately one pound); at 4 months, the increase was 0.1 kg (approximately three ounces), and thereafter mean weight in both groups at every assessment was lower (but not significantly) than pre-treatment.

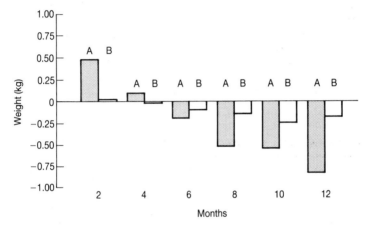

Figure 7.2   Differences in mean weight as compared to pre-treatment during therapy with Premarin (conjugated equine oestrogens ▨) or placebo ☐. Treatment A: Premarin for 6 months, then placebo for 6 months; treatment B: placebo for 6 months, then Premarin for 6 months. (From Campbell S, Whitehead M I 1977 In: Greenblatt R B, Studd J W W (eds) Clinics in obstetrics and gynaecology. W B Saunders, London and Philadelphia 4 (1): pp 31–47. Reproduced with permission.)

The authors concluded that gross weight gain which followed administration of exogenous oestrogens was more likely due to gluttony. However, two caveats must be added. The above data relate to administration of unopposed oestrogens and the effects of progestogen addition must be considered. Secondly, the data are expressed as mean values for the entire group. This does not exclude a sub-group of women who might exhibit marked increases in weight.

Many studies of combined oestrogen/progestogen therapy have investigated weight change. The majority report no significant increase in mean weight. However, again, this does not exclude a small, susceptible sub-group which experiences dramatic weight gain. There can be no doubt that a small minority of women claim weight increases in excess of 3–4 kg within a few weeks of starting HRT. Various explanations are available. Fluid retention is one but, in our experience, cannot be common because the weight that has been gained so rapidly is not usually lost if HRT is stopped. Rarely, progestogen addition appears to cause fluid retention and weight gain. In this circumstance, these problems occur only during the oestrogen/progestogen phase of treatment and resolve in the oestrogen-only part of therapy. Anecdotally, such women tend to have experienced identical problems premenstrually during the reproductive era.

An alternative explanation is that oestrogens, in some women, stimulate the appetite. It is not known whether this might be a direct effect or mediated through changes in mood. Poor appetite can be associated with depressed mood which may be improved by HRT (see Question 4.7). Paradoxically, mood elevation in some women by HRT results in weight loss because they stop 'comfort eating'. Yet another explanation is that HRT is associated with weight gain because of a change in the smoking habit. Many doctors appear to have concerns about use of HRT by tobacco-users (see Question 5.37 and Table 5.2). Therefore, HRT may be prescribed upon the condition that the patient either reduces or stops smoking. In this circumstance, we have observed dramatic weight gain which often exceeds 6–7 kg in 2–3 months. In this type of patient, stopping HRT is not followed by weight loss.

Thus, while some patients report dramatic weight increases when starting HRT (and others report decreases), the currently available literature clearly indicates that HRT does not cause significant weight gain in the majority of women.

7.4 Does HRT cause hypertension?

This is discussed in Question 9.48.

7.5 What are the symptoms of oestrogen over-dosage?

In our experience, these are significant breast tenderness, nipple sensitivity, leg cramps, nausea and fluid retention. They occur more commonly in perimenopausal women because of surges in endogenous ovarian activity (see Questions 5.16 and 5.18), and also in the woman who is many years postmenopausal and who has just started HRT. Gradual, stepwise increases in oestrogen dose in the latter group are discussed in Question 6.28. In an early postmenopausal woman (within 2–5 years of menopause) the occurrence of these symptoms and their continuation for more than 6−8 weeks after initiation of HRT would be an indication to consider a reduction in the oestrogen dose.

7.6 Does the route of administration affect the frequency/nature of side-effects?

Only to a small extent. The side-effects reported in Tables 7.1 and 7.2, and the problem of weight gain which some women allege results from use of HRT, can arise with all routes of administration. However, some symptoms occur only or largely with certain routes of administration.

Oral administration

Dyspepsia or gastrointestinal symptoms appear to occur in 3−4% of women taking oral oestrogens. Sometimes, these can be abolished or minimized by taking the tablet with food and/or at bedtime, rather than in the morning. If these strategies are unsuccessful then a non-oral route should be considered.

Rarely, once daily administration fails to control vasomotor symptoms effectively for the 24 hours until administration of the next tablet. This loss of response is likely to be due to a fall in plasma oestrogen values which may occur towards the end of the 24-hour period after tablet ingestion. Thus, tablet taking in the morning results in flushes waking the patient in the early hours of the following morning; taking the tablet at bedtime results in flushes arising early during the following evening. Twice daily administration of the oestrogen usually solves this problem.

Failure to absorb orally administered oestrogens from the gastrointestinal tract is considered in Question 9.34.

Transdermal administration

The problem of skin irritation with oestradiol patches is discussed in Question 6.12.

Poor adhesion which results in the patch falling off is a potential problem. The patches are waterproof and therefore should remain in place during bathing and showering. However, some patients report that the patch persistently falls off in water. In this situation, we advise that the patches be removed prior to bathing and applied to the backing membrane which comes with the patch. The patch can then be reapplied to the skin after bathing when the skin is quite dry.

Intra-vaginal administration

The potential problems of systemic absorption due to excessive use of oestrogen creams in the patient and her partner are discussed in Questions 6.23 and 6.24.

Subcutaneous administration

Infrequently, the implant site may become infected and the implant is sometimes extruded. This appears to occur more commonly if implantation causes a small haematoma due, presumably, to bleeding into the subcutaneous tissues. We have not seen these problems reported in the medical literature and do not know the incidence. To try to minimize these problems, we use a suture to close the skin wound (which the patient removes 5 days later) and apply a pressure dressing which the patient removes 4-6 hours after implantation.

Very rarely, patients complain of tenderness on direct pressure (usually with intercourse) over the site of a previous implant inserted into the lower, anterior abdominal wall. A small mass is easily palpable. Indeed, numerous tiny masses can often be felt and resemble a subcutaneous 'necklace'. We suspect that these represent fibrosis around the implants. Avoidance of local pressure is all that is required.

PROGESTOGENS

There can be no doubt that most problems with combined oestrogen/ progestogen HRT stem from the progestogen component. Rather surprisingly, very scant data on the precise nature, incidence and severity of these side-effects are available. The reasons for this are that few comparative studies have investigated the symptomatic and psychological impact of doses of progestogens which are protective to the endometrium. We question the relevance of determining the consequences of adding a dosage of progestogen which is greatly in excess of that required for endometrial protection. Additionally, the few studies that have been performed have investigated study groups comprising, for the most part, between 15 and 50 patients. There is some agreement that while the majority of patients are not affected adversely by the progestogen a minority do experience significant side-effects.

7.7 Is it possible to predict those women who will experience significant progestogenic side-effects?

Sparse data are available but they concur with our clinical experience.

Women who have experienced problematic premenstrual syndrome (PMS) during the reproductive era appear more likely to suffer problems with progestogens when added to oestrogens postmenopausally. It has been suggested that such women should be considered hormonally (and in particular progestogen) 'vulnerable'. Few data are available at this time because confirmation that PMS-sufferers are more likely to have menopausal problems requires longitudinal studies of large numbers of women. It is not clear whether the link, if one exists, between PMS and menopausal problems is in part hormonal, in part due to expectations, or to a combination of these factors.

7.8 What adverse effects can progestogens cause?

These can be physical or psychological; numerous side-effects have been attributed to progestogens and those that we encounter most frequently are shown in Table 7.3. Because too few data on the frequency and severity of the symptoms are available for meaningful conclusions, they are presented in alphabetical order.

Table 7.3 Physical and psychological side-effects associated with administration of progestogen

Physical	Psychological
Abdominal 'cramps'	Aggression
Accident-prone	Anxiety
Acne	Apathy
Backache	Confusion
Breast tenderness	Depressed mood
Clumsiness	Difficulty making decisions
Dizziness	Emotionally labile
Flatulence	Forgetfulness
Fluid retention	Irrational
Generalized aches and pains	Irritability
Greasy skin	Panic attacks
Headaches	Poor concentration
Hot flushes	Restlessness
Poor sleep	Tearfulness
Tiredness	
Weight gain	

7.9 Is the frequency and severity of progestogenic side-effects dose-related?

The few studies that have addressed this aspect report dose-dependency. For example, as compared to placebo, the addition of norethisterone 5 mg/day for 7 days each month to women receiving oestradiol implants was associated with statistically significant adverse effects on aspects of pain (including headache and backache); concentration (including forgetfulness, confusion, difficulty in concentrating and clumsiness); behavioural change (including avoidance of work and social activities); water retention (including weight gain and breast engorgement/tenderness), and negative affect (including anxiety, restlessness, irritability, emotional lability and depression). However, in a similar placebo-controlled study, the addition of norethisterone 2.5 mg/day did not cause statistically significant changes in symptomatology or behaviour.

Because the results from the few studies which have investigated the physical and psychological effects of progestogens have been presented as means for the entire study group, it is not possible to state with confidence whether dosage reduction preferentially lowers the frequency of these adverse effects more than the severity, whether the converse applies, or whether both are reduced. In clinical practice it is our experience that dosage reduction will abolish the presence of progestogenic side-effects in some women, will reduce them to an acceptable level in others but will be completely ineffective in a minority of women.

7.10 What is the management of women with adverse progestogenic side-effects?

The various strategies can be summarized thus:

1. reducing dose
2. changing to another progestogen
3. reducing the duration of progestogen administration
4. prescribing oestrogen therapy without a progestogen, and
5. hysterectomy.

Dosage Reduction

One of the four combined, oestrogen/progestogen packs currently available (Cyclo-Progynova® 1 mg/day and 2 mg/day) contains a progestogen at a dose (norgestrel 500 μg/day) higher than that required for endometrial protection in the majority of women (see Question 6.35 and Table 6.5). Thus, if the progestogen in Cyclo-Progynova® causes undesirable effects then the dose can be reduced by the physician either prescribing another combined oestrogen/progestogen therapy with a lower daily dose of norgestrel (e.g. Prempak-C®) or by continuing to prescribe Progynova® and by adding a lower dose of norgestrel [made up from Neogest® (see Question 6.35 and Table 6.5)] preferably for 12 days each calendar month.

Changing to another progestogen

The advantages of the flexibility gained from prescribing the oestrogen and progestogen separately are discussed in Question 6.40. Certain progestogenic side-effects appear related to chemical structure |and therefore progestogen class (see Question 6.31)|. For example, acne, greasy skin and hair are, in our experience, reported more frequently with the testosterone derivatives, norethisterone and norgestrel. All combined oestrogen/progestogen packs currently available in the UK contain one of these progestogens. Changing to a progesterone derivative (medroxyprogesterone acetate or dydrogesterone) may overcome these problems. The recommended doses of various progestogens for addition to oral/transdermal oestrogen therapies are presented in Table 6.5.

With other progestogenic side-effects, for example, breast tenderness or depressed mood, the response to a change in progestogen is difficult to predict. For reasons that are not understood, switching from a norgestrel to a norethisterone-based preparation may result in abolition of the unwanted effects, but it may not. Identical comments apply to a change from a testosterone-derivative to a progesterone-derivative, and also to a change within the progestogen class, e.g. from medroxyprogesterone acetate to dydrogesterone or vice versa. Because the response to a particular progestogen cannot be predicted, it is always worthwhile changing the progestogen provided that the patient understands and accepts that success cannot be guaranteed.

As indicated previously (see Question 6.37) only sparse data are available on the recommended daily doses of various progestogens for addition to oestradiol implant therapy. Because implants tend to result in higher plasma oestradiol values than oral or transdermal therapies (see Question 6.16), we would recommend that the higher doses of the various progestogens shown in Table 6.5 be added in patients on implant therapy. Furthermore, because with oral and transdermal oestrogens the day of onset of the withdrawal bleeding can predict the underlying endometrial status (see Question 9.30 and Fig. 9.3) and a similar correlation may apply with oestradiol implants, we would suggest that the response to bleeding starting too early during the phase of progestogen addition should be an increase in progestogen dose (see also Question 6.37).

In our experience, changing the progestogen sometimes two or three times will eventually yield success in the majority of women. Those who are intolerant of all progestogens, when prescribed for 12−13 days each calendar month/cycle, have one of the following three alternatives.

Reducing the duration of progestogen addition

Some women can tolerate unwanted progestogenic effects for 7–10 days each month, but no longer. This has led to the recommendation that progestogens be added for this shorter duration. This, we believe, is acceptable provided that both the patient and the clinician remain aware that endometrial safety is being traded off against patient acceptability of the progestational agent. Seven days of progestogen addition each month is associated with a 4% incidence of endometrial hyperplasia, and 10 days with a 2% incidence.

Prescribing the oestrogen alone, without a progestogen

Progestogens are prescribed for endometrial protection. The problems which follow use of unopposed oestrogen therapy are described in Question 8.32. Such women should be aware that annual endometrial biopsy may be recommended irrespective of the presence or absence of bleeding, and that relatively short periods of use of unopposed oestrogens have been associated with an increase in risk of endometrial cancer which continues for many years after such treatment is withdrawn (see Question 8.32 and Table 8.3). Currently, no strategies exist for screening women exposed to unopposed oestrogens for endometrial cancer following the discontinuation of treatment.

Hysterectomy

In the tiny minority of women who are intolerant of all progestogens yet who require long-term oestrogen therapy, either to relieve severe, chronic symptoms (especially vaginal dryness, vasomotor disturbances or depressed mood) or to prevent against further skeletal deterioration in the presence of early osteoporosis, hysterectomy should be considered. This may sound dramatic yet there can be no doubt that hysterectomy can beneficially influence quality of life by eliminating that 7–12 days each month of ill-health caused by progestogen addition, or the anxieties about endometrial disease experienced by those women taking unopposed oestrogens.

8. Risks and contraindications

Concerns about the safety of HRT are frequently cited by doctors and patients alike as a reason for not prescribing or taking it. Much of this concern is misplaced and often is based on data relating to the contraceptive pill which, as we have already stressed, cannot and should not be extrapolated to HRT.

We will classify safety concerns as either 'risks' or 'contraindications'. A risk is the likelihood of a condition developing as a direct result of treatment. With HRT this, by and large, refers to the risk of cancer. A contraindication is a condition which is likely to be exacerbated or aggravated by taking HRT. Circumstances in which HRT should not be prescribed (except by very specialized menopause clinics) are termed 'absolute' contraindications (Table 8.1). 'Relative' contraindications are situations in which HRT can usually be prescribed, but careful assessment may be required before commencing treatment and only certain types of treatment or routes of administration may be advisable. Although the term 'relative' contraindication may be a misnomer, we use it to draw a distinction between those conditions where the primary care physician may prescribe and the absolute contraindications where, we believe, expert opinion should be sought.

We wish to stress that some of our attitudes to use of HRT in patients with absolute and relative contraindications differ from the information provided by the manufacturers in the Data Sheets for their HRT preparations. We suspect that some of this information has been extrapolated from experience with the contraceptive pill and, for reasons discussed elsewhere (see Question 6.2), such an extrapolation may be invalid — particularly with regard to thrombotic disease. Our attitudes are based on experience with HRT preparations.

Table 8.1 Absolute contraindications to hormone replacement therapy

Endometrial cancer
Breast cancer
Known or suspected pregnancy
Undiagnosed abnormal vaginal bleeding
Severe, active liver disease with abnormal liver function tests

CONTRAINDICATIONS

8.1 In what situations should HRT not be prescribed?

Patients who are known to have, or who have had, endometrial or breast cancer are usually advised not to take HRT. Both these tumours may be responsive to oestrogens, whether endogenous or exogenous. However, there are no data in the literature which show an increased risk of recurrence in patients with such conditions who are subsequently prescribed HRT. The converse also applies because the required studies have not been performed. Until they are, HRT is best avoided in such patients unless expert advice is obtained. Alternative strategies for treating these patients are discussed in Question 8.27.

Pregnancy may cause amenorrhoea in the perimenopausal woman and if this is suspected then it should be excluded by the appropriate investigations. Spontaneous ovarian activity and ovulation may recur after many months of ovarian inactivity in perimenopausal women and carry a risk of pregnancy. Unfortunately, many women regard the onset of irregular menstruation as signifying the end of fertility and consequently they discontinue contraceptive methods. The importance of continuing with contraception for at least 12 months after menopause if the patient is aged 50 years or over, or for at least 24 months after menopause if this occurred under age 50 years, should be stressed. Contraception in perimenopausal women is discussed further in Chapter 12. If HRT was taken in error during the early stages of pregnancy we think it unlikely that the low plasma levels of oestrogen and progestogen achieved with standard HRT preparations would have an adverse effect on the developing fetus. However, there are no data to support this belief and it can be argued that the more androgenic progestogens (norgestrel and norethisterone) could have a virilizing effect on the developing fetus if taken at a critical phase of organogenesis. Consequently, if pregnancy is suspected HRT must not be prescribed until this has been excluded.

A history of postmenopausal bleeding (an episode of vaginal bleeding more than 12 months after the last menstrual period), of inter-menstrual or post-coital bleeding, or of abnormally heavy periods in the perimenopausal patient demands appropriate investigation before commencing HRT. This usually requires a pelvic examination, cervical smear, and dilatation and curettage (D&C) or endometrial biopsy as a minimum. There is a small but well recognised incidence of endometrial hyperplasia and carcinoma in untreated women, and it is vital that such patients are identified and treated accordingly before HRT is prescribed. Otherwise, use of HRT may lead to a rapid progression of the endometrial disease (see also Questions 8.21 and 9.15).

8.2 What about women with hypertension?

In general, this is not considered a contraindication to HRT, although for reasons explained in more detail in Question 9.48 the non-oral route of administration may be preferable. However, if hypertension is first detected during the initial pre-treatment examination then it should be investigated and brought under control before HRT is commenced. Similarly, if the blood pressure is poorly controlled in a known hypertensive, then better control should be attempted before commencing HRT.

8.3 Is it safe to prescribe HRT to a woman with a strong family history of hypertension?

Yes. Such a woman may develop hypertension whether or not she takes HRT, and currently there is no evidence that HRT increases this risk further. This is discussed in more detail in Question 9.48.

8.4 What should be done if a woman develops hypertension while taking HRT?

This is fully discussed in Question 9.48.

8.5 Is it safe to prescribe HRT to women with a strong family history of ischaemic heart disease?

Yes. The reduced risk of cardiovascular disease with HRT has already been fully discussed (see Questions 4.32 and 5.37). Women with a family history of ischaemic heart disease may be at an increased risk from angina and myocardial infarction but our current understanding is that they will derive the same benefits from HRT as compared with women without a relevant family history. Indeed, HRT may be one of the best preventative treatments available for them. However, it is important that preventable or correctable risk factors are not overlooked. Thus, appropriate investigations, such as a lipid profile, should be performed and the appropriate advice regarding diet, smoking and weight should be given.

As discussed in Question 4.33, all routes of oestrogen administration reduce total cholesterol levels principally through a suppression of the low density lipoprotein (LDL)-cholesterol fraction which is atherogenic. However, oral and non-oral therapies have quite different effects on plasma triglyceride, which some authorities believe is an independent risk factor for ischaemic heart disease. Oral therapies elevate plasma triglyceride levels whereas non-oral therapies do not. Thus, all routes of oestrogen administration are appropriate for patients with familial hypercholesterolaemia; however, it seems sensible to prescribe non-oral oestrogens to patients with familial hypertriglyceridaemia.

The onset of menopausal symptoms often makes women seek medical advice for the first time since the birth of their last child, perhaps many years previously. Consequently, attendance at a menopause clinic provides an ideal opportunity to re-examine the family history and to determine the presence of risk factors which may have developed or changed during the previous 10-20 years.

8.6 What about a woman who already has angina or who has had a myocardial infarction?

Previously, these women have been considered as being unsuitable for HRT. However, because of the proven benefit of HRT on ischaemic heart disease this stance appears paradoxical. In one American study the incidence of fatal myocardial infarction was observed to be 50% lower in women with a previous myocardial infarction or angina who had taken HRT, as compared to those women with a similar history who had not taken oestrogens (see Question 5.37 and Table 5.2). A similar protective effect was observed in women with a history of hypertension. Thus, HRT does not increase the risk of further, fatal ischaemic heart disease in these women; indeed, it reduces it. Consequently, HRT is not contraindicated in women with a history of myocardial infarction or hypertension. Indeed, the data suggest that women with these problems should be offered HRT to reduce the later risk of fatal myocardial infarction.

8.7 Can I prescribe HRT to a woman who has had a previous deep vein thrombosis?

Much of the evidence on the effect of oestrogens on coagulation and fibrinolytic factors is based on experience with the contraceptive pill. It is well established that ethinyl oestradiol may cause adverse changes in such factors but, as discussed in Question 6.2, these data should not be extrapolated to HRT. The synthetic oestrogens prescribed in contraceptive formulations are more potent than the natural oestrogens prescribed in HRT with respect to hepatic markers (see Question 6.2 and Table 6.2).

There is a consensus that pill administration causes changes in fibrinolytic and coagulation factors. The majority of studies of HRT have reported no such changes; one or two studies of oral HRT have reported that natural oestrogens adversely affect fibrinolytic/coagulation mechanisms, but the spectrum and severity of changes are less than those observed with the pill.

Epidemiological data on the incidence of venous thrombotic disease in oral HRT-users are relatively sparse, but no increase in incidence has been noted in the few studies that have been performed. Thus, it seems unlikely that the low doses of oestrogen used in oral HRT cause clinically relevant fibrinolytic and coagulation changes. However, any potential effect will be related not only to the dose of oestrogen but also, perhaps, to the route of administration. With oral treatment a 'bolus' of oestrogen passes to the liver via the portal vein after absorption of the steroid from the gastrointestinal tract (see Question 6.6). This does not occur with non-orally administered oestrogens. Consequently, in women with risk factors for venous thrombosis a non-oral route seems preferable, but we stress that this is hypothetical at present.

There are a number of considerations which must be taken into account when assessing a patient with a history of deep vein thrombosis. For example, we believe that it is important to distinguish between a thrombosis associated with a recognized risk factor, such as a prolonged period of immobilization (post-partum, post-traumatic), or post-operatively (especially after pelvic surgery), from the thrombosis which occurred 'spontaneously' with no obvious risk factor(s) present. In the former group, the thrombosis may be related solely to the risk factor and while the risk of a second thrombosis is increased (because of the previous thrombosis), it may not rise further because of use of HRT. In the latter group in which 'spontaneous' venous thrombosis appears to have occurred, there may be an inherent abnormality of fibrinolysis or coagulation. We believe that in this group such an abnormality should be excluded before HRT is commenced. If such an abnormality is identified then an expert haematological opinion should be sought.

The second consideration is the interval between the venous thrombotic event and the menopause. Not uncommonly, we see women who experienced a deep venous thrombosis (DVT) in their early 20s or 30s; who then menstruated regularly until their late 40s, and who subsequently requested HRT for relief of symptoms in their early 50s. Because of the previous DVT, HRT was withheld. This is illogical. The average daily plasma oestradiol value achieved during the normal ovulatory cycle in the reproductive era is higher than that achieved with oral and transdermal HRT (see Question 6.5 and Fig. 6.1). Therefore, why let a woman be exposed to her own ovarian function and then withhold HRT? If oestrogens were such a potent cause of venous thrombotic disease then the risk of further DVT would be increased around ovulation, the time of maximal oestradiol production in the non-pregnant woman. This does not happen. Furthermore, many of these women will have had a normal pregnancy and puerperium between the DVT and the menopause. We would argue that the risk of a further DVT is much greater during pregnancy when marked changes in fibrinolysis and coagulation occur than it is with HRT.

Yet another consideration is the criteria employed to diagnose the original venous thrombotic event. All too often the history is inconclusive and the diagnosis was made solely by physical examination which is known to be unreliable. In patients with a 'history of DVT' we have performed venograms and found these to be quite normal.

There are patients who present with a quite different history in whom we are concerned about prescribing HRT. These include women developing apparently spontaneous venous thrombosis, appropriately diagnosed, late during the climacteric or early postmenopausal years. Post-thrombosis, there has been no exposure to normal ovarian function and therefore the effects of plasma oestradiol levels of approximately 200–400 mol/l (the values usually achieved with oral and transdermal HRT) have not been tested. We also have concerns about women who developed a proven DVT early in pregnancy (especially if recurrent), or soon after starting the oral contraceptive pill. We would argue that in these situations the rate of rise of plasma oestradiol levels might be more important than the absolute levels achieved in causing fibrinolytic/coagulation changes.

Every woman who has had one DVT is at an increase in risk of a further thrombotic episode, whether she takes HRT or not. In those groups in whom we have expressed concern we offer a pre-treatment coagulation profile.

8.8 What fibrinolytic/coagulation tests should be requested?

This will depend on the advice and recommendation of the local haematologist. However, these should include measures of both the extrinsic system (i.e. prothrombin time) and the intrinsic system (KCCT). Anti-thrombin III is a particularly important factor which inactivates thrombin and a significant reduction ($>20\%$) in this factor has been found to be highly predictive of sub-clinical venous thromboembolic disease. Anti-thrombin III may be reduced by as much as 11% with synthetic oestrogens, such as ethinyl oestradiol, but in the same study conjugated equine oestrogens 1.25 mg/day had no suppressive effect. This again illustrates the importance of differentiating between the various types of oestrogens when considering risks of thromboembolic disease. Protein S and C levels, if available, are also helpful to exclude underlying coagulation defects.

8.9 Does the same apply if the patient, in addition, has a history of pulmonary embolism?

Yes, provided the source of the embolus was thought to be a DVT. A distinction between those thrombotic episodes associated with recognized risk factors and those occurring spontaneously should be made and treatment or investigations initiated as above (see Question 8.8).

8.10 Is HRT contraindicated in a woman with varicose veins?

No. The concern about oestrogens and varicose veins stems from the erroneous assumption that the presence of varicose veins increases the risk of deep vein thrombosis. Because no such association exists, there seems no reason to deny HRT to women with varicose veins.

8.11 Can a woman with a history of superficial thrombophlebitis (or phlebothrombosis) be given HRT?

Yes. These are superficial problems and are not associated with deep vein thrombosis. HRT with natural oestrogens does not appear to increase the risk of these conditions. Soon after starting treatment a patient may complain of leg pains but these tend to be bilateral and are not related to venous thrombotic disease (see Question 7.2).

8.12 Is it safe to prescribe HRT to a heavy smoker?

Yes. As discussed above, there is no increase in the risk of fatal myocardial infarction in patients with a history of hypertension, stroke and ischaemic heart disease with HRT. One epidemiological study from the USA has reported no significant difference in the incidence of acute fatal myocardial infarction in heavy smokers who had used oestrogens as compared to those who had not taken HRT. This contrasts with the protective effect shown for women with other risk factors for myocardial infarction (see Question 5.37 and Table 5.2). This suggests that the beneficial effects of oestrogens on cardiovascular disease risk are negated by tobacco use. However, there is no reason to deny HRT to tobacco users.

8.13 Can overweight women be given HRT, and if so, are there any precautions?

On current evidence, the arterial risks associated with obesity are not worsened by the administration of HRT, and thus obese women can take oestrogens. Obese postmenopausal women tend to have higher circulating oestrone levels than their counterparts of normal weight. This is a result of the increased peripheral conversion of androstenedione to oestrone in adipose tissue (see Question 2.4). Consequently, they may suffer with fewer symptoms and, in general, tend to have a lower risk of osteoporosis although weight itself cannot be regarded as an accurate predictor of those who might develop this condition.

The lack of overall effect of HRT on weight is discussed in Question 7.3.

8.14 Is it safe to prescribe HRT to a patient with multiple risk factors for cardiovascular disease or thrombosis, i.e. an overweight smoker with angina?

Yes, but HRT may have less beneficial effects on her life expectancy than an alteration in her smoking and dietary habits, and treatment of her angina. Nevertheless, HRT may lead to some reduction in risk.

8.15 Can diabetics be given HRT?

Yes. There is no reason why these women should not be given HRT. Diabetics, particularly those with juvenile onset diabetes, are at an increased risk of cardiovascular and peripheral vascular disease.

Both oestrogens and progestogens affect carbohydrate metabolism and thus, the diabetic control must be monitored very closely during the first few months of treatment and may require adjustment. In summary, the high dose oestrogen/progestogen combinations used in oral contraceptives have been shown to have adverse effects on carbohydrate metabolism. However, the lower more 'physiological' doses of oestrogens used in HRT seem to affect glucose tolerance less. Furthermore, differences in response have been observed with different routes of oestrogen administration. In normal women, oral oestrogens increase plasma glucose levels more than non-orally administered oestrogens. It is not clear whether similar differences occur in diabetics but, if they do, then a non-oral route of administration would seem preferable in patients with abnormal carbohydrate metabolism.

Progestogens have numerous effects upon glucose tolerance. However, the effects of combined oestrogen/progestogen therapies used in HRT on carbohydrate metabolism have not been studied extensively, and it is not clear whether the addition of a low dose of progestogen in a sequential fashion to the oestrogen will be relevant clinically. Because of the uncertainty about the exact nature and magnitude of any change, no adjustment to the insulin regimen need be made initially. However, glucose levels should be monitored closely and the insulin dosage adjusted according to the response.

8.16 Is liver disease a contraindication to HRT?

This will depend upon the nature and the severity of the liver disease.

In the presence of severe active liver disease (with abnormal liver function tests), we believe that HRT should be withheld. This is based on the assumption that it is undesirable to present a further metabolic load to a diseased organ; the majority of oestrogen is degraded and metabolized within the liver. However, we stress that no data are available on the effects of HRT upon liver function in such women. If HRT is prescribed then, at least in theory, administration of oestrogen by a non-oral route would reduce the risk of compromising the liver further by avoiding the 'bolus' of oestrogen achieved with oral therapy.

In women who have mild liver disease with only slightly abnormal liver function tests, or who have had liver disease which has resolved completely, there seems no reason why HRT should not be prescribed. However, in these women it may be advisable to use a non-oral route of administration as discussed above.

In conditions such as Gilbert's syndrome in which there is only minimal disturbance of liver function HRT is not contraindicated and either the oral or non-oral route of administration can be used. The relationships between liver disease and HRT are considered further in Question 9.54.

8.17 Can a patient with gallstones have HRT?

Oral, natural oestrogens can cause a change in the composition of bile which may lead to an increase in risk of gallstones. Thus, in women known to have gallstones or gall bladder disease HRT should be prescribed with caution.

One case report has observed less changes in bile composition with transdermal oestradiol than with oral therapy. It is possible that the non-oral route may be a better alternative for such patients, but further data are required before this can be widely recommended.

After a patient has had her gallstones removed she may use HRT again.

8.18 Can a woman with fibroids be given HRT, and if so, what is likely to happen to the fibroids?

Fibroids are very common, are often asymptomatic, and frequently are diagnosed for the first time on routine pelvic examination. However, they are oestrogen-dependent and may enlarge with HRT. The majority of these will cause no problems but some may result in heavy withdrawal bleeding and others may achieve a considerable size (see Question 9.41). The risk of malignant change is less than 1%.

Women with small, asymptomatic fibroids, therefore, should not be precluded from taking HRT but we would recommend regular monitoring with an annual pelvic examination and also, perhaps, with pelvic ultrasound, as indicated. The management of patients with large fibroids or those causing heavy withdrawal bleeding is discussed in Question 9.41.

8.19 Can a woman who has had endometriosis take HRT, and what is the risk of recurrence?

This problem is discussed fully in Question 9.45. In summary, endometriotic tissue can respond to oestrogens, even if many years have elapsed between menopause and starting HRT. However, the possible risks of a recurrence of endometriosis must be balanced against the benefits of HRT. Often women with severe endometriosis have undergone a surgically induced menopause (bilateral oophorectomy), and thus are in special need of HRT to reduce their risk of future cardiovascular disease and osteoporosis (see Questions 5.4–5.13). In women in whom all endometriotic tissue has been removed at surgery, the chances of recurrence appear lower than if endometriotic tissue had been left behind. However, even with apparent complete surgical removal of all endometriotic tissue, we have seen the disease reactivated with HRT. This may be because endometriosis can arise de novo from coelomic metaplasia; or because microscopic disease, not visible to the naked eye, remained after surgery. In women with residual disease after surgery, it is often recommended that HRT be withheld for at least 9 months after surgery and then commenced. However, we have seen the disease reactivated in women starting HRT 10 years after menopause (see Question 9.45).

It is not possible to generalize further and each case has to be judged on its merits. We believe that endometriosis probably poses one of the most difficult treatment decisions. Primary care physicians should not hesitate to seek specialist advice if they are in any doubt as to whether or not to prescribe for these women.

8.20 What is the best way to prescribe HRT for patients with previous endometriosis?

The optimal treatment regimen is not known. In terms of overall stimulation by the oestrogen, there would not appear to be any differences between oral and non-oral routes at comparable doses. However, we would advise against using sustained release preparations, such as oestradiol implants, as first-line treatment. These can result in higher plasma oestradiol values and they cannot be discontinued quickly should symptoms indicative of recurrence develop (see Question 9.45). Frequently, women with a history of severe endometriosis will have undergone hysterectomy and therefore, under normal circumstances, would not require progestogens (see Question 8.39). However, the underlying pathophysiology of endometriosis is oestrogenic activation of ectopic endometrial tissue. Progestogens have an antimitotic, suppressant effect upon the endometrium, so, in theory, it may be advisable to add a progestogen to the oestrogen in a continuous daily fashion. We stress that this strategy is hypothetical and confirmatory data are not available.

8.21 What is endometrial hyperplasia and is it a contraindication to HRT?

Hyperplasia literally means overgrowth of the endometrium and is usually characterized by an increase in the activity of the epithelial glandular elements of the endometrium. Hyperplasia is a pre-malignant condition and is usually divided into two main types. Both are believed to result from chronic, unopposed oestrogen stimulation.

1. Cystic glandular hyperplasia. This is illustrated in Figure 8.1. It is the more benign form and the risk of subsequent malignant change is probably less than 1%. The glands can assume various appearances; when widely dilated they resemble 'Swiss cheese'. Biochemically, cystic glandular hyperplasia appears to behave in a similar fashion to normal proliferative endometrium.

2. Atypical hyperplasia. This is illustrated in Figure 8.2. It is a more sinister condition and carries a much higher risk of subsequent malignant change. The rate varies from approximately 10–15% with mild atypia, through to 25% with moderate disease and to 50% with severe atypical hyperplasia in studies of relatively short follow-up. Much longer-term studies (of approximately 10 years' duration) have reported a 100% progression of severe atypical hyperplasia to carcinoma.

Atypical hyperplasia is usually characterized by nuclear atypia, pseudostratification and gland crowding with 'back to back' gland formation. Biochemically, it appears to be an abnormal tissue with an

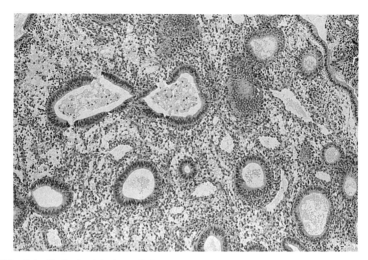

Fig. 8.1 Cystic glandular hyperplasia: note numerous dilated glands.

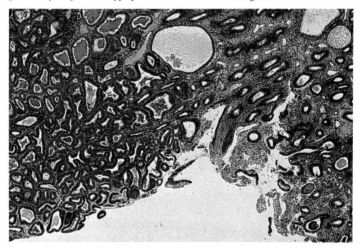

Fig. 8.2 Atypical hyperplasia: note pseudostratification and gland crowding.

exaggerated response to oestrogenic stimulation. Because of the higher rate of malignant change (and because this may take many years to develop), we believe that hysterectomy should be seriously considered with this condition.

The need for a routine pre-treatment endometrial biopsy before commencing HRT is discussed in Question 9.15. In women previously diagnosed as having cystic hyperplasia we believe that a follow-up biopsy should be performed approximately 4−6 months after starting combined HRT to confirm that the endometrium has reversed to normal. The progestogen should be prescribed at adequate daily dose and for an adequate duration each month/cycle, at least for 12 days and perhaps even longer (some authorities recommend up to 21 days each month). Failure of an adequate progestational stimulus to reverse the hyperplasia should raise the question of hysterectomy.

We believe that if atypical hyperplasia is diagnosed then hysterectomy is advisable before commencing HRT. After the endometrium is removed there is no further risk and HRT can be prescribed.

8.22 Can a woman with migraine be given HRT?

The relationship between HRT and migraine is fully discussed in Question 9.56.

8.23 Is otosclerosis an absolute contraindication to HRT?

Otosclerosis is a condition characterized by progressive irreversible deafness which appears to worsen during pregnancy. There are no published studies on the effects of HRT, and the only evidence we have is anecdotal. In our experience, we have seen two patients with otosclerosis who were prescribed HRT and their hearing deteriorated within a few weeks of starting treatment. However, we are aware of other doctors who have prescribed HRT to women with otosclerosis and no change in the hearing has occurred. Thus, it is impossible to make specific recommendations but we would urge caution when considering prescribing to such women. The advice of an ENT specialist may be helpful.

8.24 What is the risk of recurrence of malignant melanoma if a woman is prescribed HRT?

Again, this is an unknown. It is well recognized that high levels of oestrogen (as in pregnancy) stimulate melanocytes as illustrated by the appearance of a linea nigra and chloasma in pregnancy, and of the latter in a small number of women taking the oral contraceptive pill. We have not seen either of these conditions in women taking oral or transdermal HRT. However, we have seen mild chloasma in a couple of patients receiving oestradiol implants.

We believe that patients should be informed of a possible, but unknown increased risk of recurrence. The decision whether or not to take HRT must be balanced between this unknown risk and the known benefits of HRT.

8.25 Is hypothyroidism a contraindication to HRT?

No. This should be treated before commencing HRT. Once the patient is euthyroid there is no reason why she cannot be given HRT.

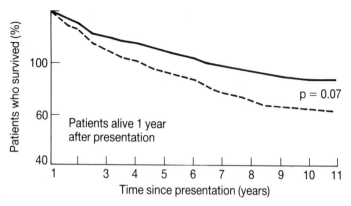

Fig. 8.3 Percentage survival in patients who had undergone surgery for ovarian cancer who received hormone replacement therapy within a year (———), versus corrected percentage survival if these patients had not received hormone replacement (- - -) within a year according to time since presentation at hospital. (From Eeles R A, Tan S, Wiltshaw E et al 1991 British Medical Journal 302: 259–262. Reproduced with permission.)

8.26 Is previous ovarian cancer a contraindication to HRT?

Very few data are available to answer this question. However, one recently published, retrospective study reported that the subsequent survival of patients with ovarian cancer who were alive one year after initial presentation and who had used HRT were slightly, but not significantly, better than non-HRT users. These results are illustrated in Figure 8.3. Further data are urgently required to confirm or refute this beneficial effect. Based upon this study, there seems no reason to withhold HRT from patients with ovarian cancer. Approximately 20% will have stage I disease which carries a 10-year survival of approximately 70%. Some of these women will be young and the physical and psychological sequelae of premature surgical menopause are likely to be considerable.

8.27 What strategies are available for women who have had endometrial or breast cancer?

As stated in Question 8.1, the risk of recurrence of these conditions with HRT is unknown. With endometrial cancer, it seems probable that the potential for recurrence with HRT will depend upon histological grading, receptor status and stage of the tumour. Each of these must be considered. For example, anaplastic tumours are not usually hormone dependent and do not contain oestradiol receptor (they are termed receptor negative). Thus, it is most unlikely that HRT will influence the risk of recurrence in any way. Conversely, well-differentiated adenocarcinomas, which are usually receptor positive, may be influenced. However, metastatic disease from a well-differentiated, primary endometrial cancer is often receptor negative and this should reduce the risk of recurrence with HRT. Similar comments are likely to apply to breast cancer.

Patients with endometrial or breast cancer have the following alternatives.

1. *Symptomatic treatment with non-hormone preparations*

These include clonidine for hot flushes, antidepressants or tranquillizers for mood changes, or agents such as vitamin B6 or oil of evening primrose which some women find helpful for mood swings and breast tenderness. Vaginal lubricants can be used for dyspareunia. The benefits of these treatments are limited but they may serve to make the symptoms more bearable in some women. These alternatives were discussed more fully in Questions 5.23 and 5.24.

2. *Prophylactic treatment with non-sex hormone preparations*

There is no alternative to HRT for reduction of arterial disease risk apart from eliminating obvious risk factors such as obesity, hypertension, hyperlipidaemia and tobacco use.

The potential role of calcitonin and the bisphosphonates as prophylactic therapy against osteoporosis was discussed in Question 5.34. In summary, calcitonin has been shown to conserve bone mass in early postmenopausal women. It has the disadvantages of being expensive and, at present, can only be given by injection. Research to try to develop a more acceptable form of administration (an intranasal aerosol) is currently under way. The bisphosphonates have been shown to conserve bone in women with established osteoporosis; they may have a role as prophylactic treatment in early postmenopausal women.

3. *Symptomatic and prophylactic treatment with progestogens*

The beneficial effects of progestational agents, by themselves, in reducing the frequency of flushing episodes were discussed fully in Question 4.5 and illustrated in Figure 4.1. There are some data that certain types of progestogens may reduce postmenopausal bone loss. It must be stressed, however, that the effects of progestogens on breast tissue are also unknown. They have been incriminated in the genesis of breast cancer in young women taking the combined, oral contraceptive pill, and some data indicate that the progestogen component may increase mitotic activity in breast epithelium. Furthermore, there are theoretical concerns that by adversely influencing lipid and lipoprotein metabolism, progestogen-only therapy might increase the risk of arterial disease.

4. Treatment with HRT

Some women experience such severe menopausal symptoms that the quality of their life is grossly disrupted and they often say that they see little point in continuing to live in this manner. In this situation (and if the above strategies have been unsuccessful), we feel that it is reasonable to offer these women low-dose HRT. This is only done after full discussion with the patient and on the clear understanding that we do not know whether HRT will or will not increase the likelihood of a recurrence of their tumour. Thus, the fully informed patient makes the decision. To verify that the patient has been adequately counselled, we make a statement to this effect in the patient's notes which we ask the patient to sign; this is witnessed by the doctor and by a third party, i.e. the clinic sister. This statement should not be interpreted as vindication of treatment. However, in this situation where the risks of HRT are unknown whereas the benefits are clearly defined, we believe that the patient has the right to choose. Many women opt for HRT frequently citing the old adage 'the quality of life is more important than the quantity', or words to that effect.

A further potential problem in such women is the reaction of the specialist overseeing the follow-up of their carcinoma, particularly breast cancer. Wherever possible, the advice and cooperation of the specialist should be sought and although some breast surgeons are adamantly against HRT it has surprised us how many are willing to sanction its use in such circumstances. In these patients referral to a specialist menopause clinic is probably advisable because it is likely to have greater experience in dealing with such problems.

RISKS

8.28 What are the principal risks of HRT?

Apart from conditions such as gallstones and otosclerosis which have been discussed above, the major concern about the risk of HRT is confined to the risk of cancer. Before discussing whether HRT has any effect or not on the incidence of certain cancers, it is essential to appreciate the background risk of that cancer in an untreated, age-matched population. Figure 8.4 shows the age-related incidence of the four female cancers most likely to be affected by HRT. There are well recognized age-related changes in the incidence of these cancers; for instance, the incidence of carcinoma of the cervix peaks in the mid-forties whereas that of ovarian carcinoma peaks in the mid-fifties, and the peak incidence of endometrial carcinoma is in the early sixties. With

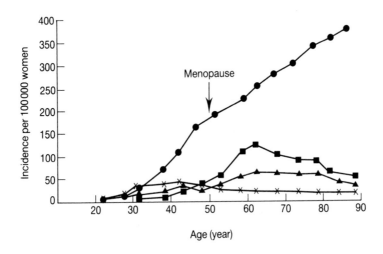

Fig. 8.4 Incidence per 100 000 women of various cancers, by age. ● = breast, ■ = endometrium, ▲ = ovary, × = cervix. (From Gambrell R D Jr 1983 Reproductive Endocrinology 1: 27–40. Reproduced with permission.)

breast cancer there is a progressive increase in risk with age, but the rate of increase varies at different ages. This is discussed in Question 8.34.

The important issue is whether or not these background increases in risk are affected by HRT. The following sections address this problem for each cancer, in turn.

8.29 Can a woman with a history of carcinoma of the cervix be given HRT?

Yes. There is no evidence that the incidence of cervical carcinoma is increased with HRT. Indeed, one epidemiological study reported that the incidence was reduced to below that of the expected rate in an untreated population. This reduction in HRT-users is more likely to have been due to increased patient surveillance rather than to a direct protective effect of HRT on the cervix.

Because the incidence of carcinoma of the cervix is not increased with HRT, the risk of recurrence is not likely to be influenced either. This is important because young women who have undergone Wertheim's hysterectomy with removal of both ovaries will be in particular need of HRT. Regular follow-up for the carcinoma should, of course, be continued but there is no requirement for additional measures on our current understanding.

8.30 Can HRT be prescribed to a patient who has had abnormal cervical smears and do her smears need repeating more often if she takes HRT?

Because HRT does not appear to be associated with an increase in risk of cervical carcinoma, it is difficult to understand how it might be associated with an increased risk of abnormal cytology. Progression from abnormal cytology to carcinoma is not likely to be affected by HRT. If an abnormal smear is reported before or during HRT this should be treated by standard procedures, and the HRT should be regarded as irrelevant.

8.31 Is there an increased risk of ovarian cancer with HRT?

Several large-scale epidemiological studies have failed to demonstrate an *overall* increase in risk of ovarian cancer in HRT-users. However, three separate reports have observed an increased incidence of endometrioid ovarian cancer in women taking HRT, and these are summarized in Table 8.2. The observed increases did not reach statistical significance and could be due to chance. The authors of the various reports also pointed out that other factors may be operating. For example, the histological diagnosis of endometrioid ovarian cancer can be difficult to make and around the time that these reports appeared it was being diagnosed more frequently because of increased recognition. Thus, the observed increases in incidence in these reports may merely reflect an increase in reporting rather than a true increase in incidence of this disease. Nevertheless, further data are needed and it is possible that there may be an increase in risk of this uncommon type of ovarian cancer with HRT.

8.32 What is the risk of endometrial cancer with unopposed oestrogens?

It is now well established that unopposed oestrogens (without progestogen) given cyclically (3 weeks on treatment, 1 week off), or continuously, increase the risk of endometrial cancer. There are three points worthy of special mention:

1. A 3–4-fold increase in the incidence of endometrial cancer has been observed within 6 months of commencing unopposed oestrogens by some authors. It is unlikely that oestrogens caused the cancer in this short time. A more likely explanation is that a pre-existing endometrial abnormality (hyperplasia) rapidly progressed to carcinoma after oestrogens were commenced, or that a pre-existing malignancy was unmasked because unopposed oestrogens caused vaginal bleeding requiring biopsy. There is a

Table 8.2 Studies reporting an increase in risk of endometrioid ovarian cancer

	Relative risk	95% confidence intervals
Cramer et al (JNCI, 1983, 71: 711)	1.6	0.9–2.9
Weiss et al (JNCI, 1982, 68: 95)	3.1	1.0–9.8
La Vecchia et al (JNCI, 1982, 69: 1207)	2.3	1.0–5.3

(JNCI, Journal of the National Cancer Institutes)

well recognized incidence of endometrial disease in previously untreated women who have not experienced abnormal bleeding (see Question 9.15). Thus, we would recommend that any woman who is going to take unopposed oestrogens should have a pre-treatment biopsy to exclude a pre-existing abnormality.

2. The increased risk of endometrial cancer with HRT is duration-dependent. However, it is not clear whether this relationship between risk and duration of administration is linear or exponential. If a linear relationship is assumed, then unopposed oestrogens increase the incidence of endometrial cancer from approximately 1 woman per 1000 women per annum observed in an untreated population to approximately 5 women per 1000 treated women per annum. It must be remembered that this increase in risk is cumulative.

3. There is an increased risk of endometrial cancer for many years after treatment with unopposed, cyclical oestrogens is discontinued. A recently published follow-up study of women who had taken unopposed oestrogens and subsequently discontinued treatment reported that 3 years of unopposed oestrogen therapy was associated with an 8·8-fold excess of risk between 2 and 14 years after stopping therapy. The excess risk in those women who had discontinued treatment more than 15 years previously was approximately six-fold. These data are shown in Table 8.3. Clearly, then, unopposed oestrogens have a prolonged 'carry-over' effect after treatment is withdrawn.

At present, there are no guidelines/recommendations as to how women previously exposed to unopposed oestrogens should be monitored. (See Questions 9.15 and 9.30)

8.33 Now that progestogens are being prescribed as part of HRT what is the risk of endometrial cancer?

Two large-scale epidemiological studies have addressed this issue and agree that the risk of endometrial cancer with opposed HRT is no greater than

Table 8.3 Age-adjusted incidence rates per 1000 women for endometrial cancer: number of cases, incidence rate and relative risk by duration of and years since cessation of unopposed, cyclic oestrogen therapy

Duration	Years since cessation	Woman–years	Number of cases	Incidence rate	Relative risk
None	No use	12 472	5	0.3	1.0
≤3	0–1	352	0	—	—
	2–14	1354	4	3.7	8.8
	15+	2776	7	2.3	6.2

(Adapted from Paganini Hill A, Ross R K, Henderson B E 1989 British Journal of Cancer 59: 445–447. Reproduced with permission.)

that in the untreated population. However, they disagree as to whether the risk with combined oestrogen/progestogen therapy is reduced to below that of an untreated population. In one study, the oestrogen/progestogen users had an incidence of endometrial cancer significantly reduced to below that of an untreated population, whereas in the other study the incidence rates were similar. Clearly, though, there is no increase in risk of endometrial cancer with combined therapies provided that the progestogen is added in adequate dose and for an adequate duration.

The issue of adequate dose and duration needs to be stressed as inadequate doses or durations may not have the same protective effect. This is discussed in more detail in Questions 6.35 and 6.36.

8.34 Is there an increased risk of breast cancer with HRT?

This is most probably the most controversial issue concerning exogenous oestrogen and progestogen use at present. Until very recently (when it was overtaken by lung cancer) breast cancer was the commonest malignancy in women. The incidence increases with age (Fig. 8.4) and approximately 1 in 12 women in the UK will develop breast cancer during their life. Thus, even a small percentage increase in risk with HRT will have a large impact on patient numbers.

The aetiology of breast cancer is multi-factorial. There is considerable evidence that it is related to ovarian, and in particular, to oestrogen status. For example, early age at menarche, obesity (high levels of endogenous oestrogen from peripheral conversion of androgens), and late age of menopause are all associated with an increased risk of breast cancer; conversely late menarche and early menopause decrease risk. The effects of premature menopause were discussed in detail in Chapter 5. The effect of menopause around age 50 years on breast cancer risk is illustrated in Figure 8.4. Although the risk continues to increase with advancing age, the *rate* of increase is reduced after menopause and this suggests a lowering of risk associated with reduced oestrogen production. Thus, it is necessary to determine whether replacement of oestrogen will reverse this trend in postmenopausal women.

A large number of epidemiological studies have tried to address this issue. Regrettably, many of the early studies were flawed for various reasons. These included small numbers of patients, insufficient data on oestrogen dose and duration of exposure, and failure to control adequately for factors known to influence breast cancer risk, such as family history, age at menarche and menopause, age at first live birth, and also to control for surveillance bias. Therefore, it is doubtful whether reliable conclusions can be drawn from these studies.

During the last 10 years a number of better-designed, case-control studies have been published together with some prospective studies. The 'control' populations in these studies were either hospital or population based., Although more carefully designed, the results are contradictory and they illustrate why no consensus currently exists.

The case-control studies are summarized in Table 8.4 and the prospective studies in Table 8.5. Some reported a slight increase in the risk of breast cancer with oestrogen use, but others did not. It might be argued that the fact that the data are so conflicting despite close analyses is reassuring; if there was a definite link between HRT and breast cancer, this should be clearly evident in the majority of the studies. However, we believe that it is likely that the discrepancy between the results of these studies really reflects the multifactorial aetiology of breast cancer and the lack of an appropriate control group properly matched to the HRT-treated women for every factor known to influence breast cancer risk. In addition to *overall* risk, it is important to establish whether there is a duration-dependent increase in risk with HRT, and whether any sub-groups of women are particularly susceptible.

8.35 Does the duration of oestrogen therapy influence breast cancer risk?

Relevant data from case-control studies are shown in Table 8.6 and from prospective studies in Table 8.7. None of the increases observed by the Centers for Disease Control in the USA (Wingo et al 1987) achieved statistical significance, nor did the results of the American National Cancer Institutes (Brinton et al 1986). However, the latter authors reported that the trend was significant. Two prospective studies (Buring et al 1987 and Mills et al 1989) reported significant increases in risk with between 5–9 and 6–10 years of HRT, respectively, but no significant increases as the duration was extended beyond 10 years.

Table 8.4 Relative risk of breast cancer in women receiving hormone replacement therapy; case-control studies.

Authors	Number of cases of breast cancer	Natural menopause	Bilateral oophorectomy	Overall
Jick et al (1980)	97	⋆ 3.4 (2.1−5.6) 90% CI	1.1	Not stated
Ross et al (1980)	138	1.4	0.8	1.1
Kelsey et al (1981)	332	0.9	0.9	Not stated
Hoover et al (1981)	345	1.3	1.5	⋆ 1.4 (1.0−2.0)
Hulka et al † (1982)	199	⋆ 1.7 (1.0−2.7) ⋆ 1.8 (1.2−2.7)	1.2 1.3	Not stated
Sherman et al (1983)	113	Not stated	Not stated	0.7
Hiatt et al (1984)	119	Not stated	0.7	Not stated
Kaufman et al (1984)	1610	1.3 (⟩10 years)	⋆ 0.5 (0.2−1.0) (⟩10 years)	0.9
Nomura et al † (1986)	161 183	Not stated Not stated	Not stated Not stated	0.9 1.1
Brinton et al (1986)	1960	1.0	1.1	1.0
La Vecchia et al (1986)	1108	Not stated	Not stated	⋆ 1.9 (1.35−2.75)
McDonald et al (1986)	183	0.8	1.3	0.7
Wingo et al (1987)	1369	0.8	1.3	1.0

⋆ Significantly different from a relative risk of 1. Figures in brackets indicate 95% confidence intervals except where stated.
† Where more than one set of risks is given, more than one set of subjects/controls were studied.
(Reproduced, with permission, by courtesy of Miss P Wood of Ciba-Geigy Pharmaceuticals; personal communication.)

Table 8.5 Relative risk (RR) of breast cancer in women receiving hormone replacement therapy; prospective studies

Authors	Number of women	Mean length of follow-up	Overall RR
Hoover et al (1976)	1891	12 years	1.3
Gambrell et al (1983)	5563	7 years	0.7
Buring et al (1987)	33 335	4 years	1.1
Hunt et al (1987)	4544	5.6 years	* 1.59 (1.18–2.1)
Bergkvist et al (1989)	23 244	5.7 years	1.1
Mills et al (1989)	20 341	6 years	* 1.39 (1.0–1.94)
Colditz et al (1990)	367 187	woman-years	*1.36 (current users) (1.11–1.67) 0.98 (past users)

* Significantly different from a relative risk of 1. Figures in brackets indicate 95% confidence intervals.
(Reproduced, with permission, by courtesy of Miss P Wood of Ciba-Geigy Pharmaceuticals; personal communication.)

Table 8.6 Effect of 5 or more years of hormone replacement therapy (HRT) on relative risk (RR) of breast cancer; case-control studies

Authors	Duration of HRT	RR+95% confidence intervals (CI) (if given)
*Hoover et al (1981)	⩾5 years	1.7
Hulka et al (1982)	⩾10 years	0.7 (community controls) 1.7 (hospital controls)
Kaufman et al (1982)	⩾10 years	1.3 (natural menopause) 0.5 (oophorectomized)
Nomura et al (1986)	⟩6 years	1.3 (Caucasians) 1.9 (Japanese)
*Brinton et al (1986)	5–9 years	1.1 (95% CI, 0.9–1.3)
	10–14 years	1.3 (95% CI, 0.9–1.6)
	15–19 years	1.2 (95% CI, 0.9–1.8)
	20+ years	1.5 (95% CI, 0.9–2.3)
Wingo et al (1987)	5–9 years	1.1 (95% CI, 0.8–1.5)
	10–14 years	0.8 (95% CI, 0.5–1.3)
	15–19 years	1.3 (95% CI, 0.6–2.6)
	20+ years	1.8 (95% CI, 0.6–5.8)

*Results of trend test were significant.
(Reproduced, with permission, by courtesy of Miss P Wood of Ciba-Geigy Pharmaceuticals; personal communication.)

Table 8.7 Effect of 5 or more years of hormone replacement therapy (HRT) on relative risk (RR) of breast cancer; prospective studies

Authors	Duration of HRT	RR + 95% CI
Hoover et al (1976)	15 years	*2.0 (95% CI, 1.1–3.4)
Buring et al (1987)	⩾5 years	1.3 (95% CI, 0.9–2.1)
	5–9 years	*1.5 (95% CI, 1.0–2.2)
	10+ years	0.9 (95% CI, 0.4–1.6)
Hunt et al (1987)	⩾6 years	3.6 (95% CI, 0.9–15.0)
Mills et al (1989)	6–10 years	*2.75 (95% CI, 1.6–4.6)
	10+ years	1.5 (95% CI, 0.9–2.5)
Colditz et al (1990)	10 years (past users)	0.7 (95% CI, 0.45–1.1)
	10-15 years	1.3 (95% CI, 0.8–2.0)

*Significantly different from a relative risk of 1. Figures in parentheses indicate 95% confidence intervals.
(Reproduced, with permission, by courtesy of Miss P Wood of Ciba-Geigy Pharmaceuticals; personal communication.)

8.36 Are there any sub-groups of women at particular risk for breast cancer with HRT?

If oestrogens increase breast cancer risk, then it is important that 'at risk' groups of women be identified. The epidemiologists appear to agree on one point, that the epidemiological data on this aspect are confusing. Some studies have reported that oestrogen use increases breast cancer risk in women with surgically proven 'benign' breast disease, but others have not. Other studies have reported the greatest increase in risk in women following natural menopause, while other studies have reported that this occurs after oophorectomy (see Table 8.4). Yet other studies have reported that the greatest increase in risk occurs in women with a family history of breast cancer, but others have not.

8.37 Does the type of HRT preparation have an effect on breast cancer risk?

It must be emphasized that nearly all the epidemiological data referred to previously were derived from the USA and consequently refer almost exclusively to unopposed conjugated equine oestrogens. Data on other oestrogen preparations are much more sparse. However, extrapolation of these data to other types of oestrogens which achieve similar plasma oestradiol levels would seem justified.

Whether data on natural oestrogens can be extrapolated to synthetic oestrogens is a completely different matter. Because of their greater potency on other oestrogen-dependent tissues such as the liver (see Question 6.2), it may not be valid to extrapolate in this way. This is especially important when interpreting some of the more recently published studies. The very recent Swedish study which attracted so much media attention reported no increase in risk of breast cancer in women taking conjugated equine oestrogens. However, in women taking 'oestradiol compounds' the risk was elevated. The latter group comprised women who had received either an oral oestradiol preparation or ethinyl oestradiol.

It is difficult, biologically, to understand why two preparations achieving similar plasma levels (conjugated equine oestrogens and oral oestradiol preparations) should cause dissimilar breast effects. Therefore, it has been suggested that the increase in risk observed by the Swedish workers in the women taking 'oestradiol compounds' was due to ethinyl oestradiol. The suspicion that ethinyl oestradiol might increase the risk of breast cancer in postmenopausal women was first raised in the UK study which was funded by the Medical Research Council. Until this issue is resolved, we believe that clinicians should be wary of studies which have included women taking ethinyl oestradiol, unless the results from the women using natural oestrogens are presented separately from those taking synthetic oestrogens. While it may appear strange that many of the European studies include women taking synthetic oestrogens when they are prescribed so infrequently today, it must be remembered that many women for these studies were recruited during the late 1970s when synthetic oestrogens were much more widely prescribed for HRT.

8.38 Can women with a previous history of benign breast disease take HRT?

There are two important issues here: firstly, the stage in her life when the woman developed benign breast disease (before or after starting HRT) and secondly, the histological type of disease. Additionally, 'benign breast disease' carries a small increase in lifetime risk of breast cancer. If a small increase is observed in such patients taking HRT it may be due more to the natural history of the disease rather than the use of HRT.

1. The results from the National Cancer Institutes in the USA showed that if the benign breast disease was first diagnosed after the patient had already started HRT then there seemed to be no increase in risk of breast cancer even if treatment was continued for more than 10 years. However, if the benign breast disease was diagnosed before commencing HRT then the subsequent risk of breast cancer was not increased with up to 10 years of therapy, but if oestrogens were continued for more than 10 years then a three-fold increase in risk was reported.

2. There appears to be some agreement that the histological type of breast disease is important in determining the lifetime risk of breast cancer. For

example, the presence of epitheliosis with atypia, and either lobular or ductal hyperplasia increases the subsequent risk of breast cancer, irrespective of whether HRT is administered or not. It is not clear whether the use of HRT will increase this predisposition further. This is discussed further in Question 9.51.

More data are urgently needed on the inter-relationships between HRT and certain types of benign breast disease.

8.39 Can a woman with a family history of breast cancer in a first degree relative take HRT?

Again, the data are conflicting. A woman with a family history of breast cancer in a first degree relative under the age of 50 years is at increased risk of breast cancer regardless of whether or not she takes HRT. Few studies have addressed the issue of whether HRT increases this risk further. One study reported a further increase in risk but this was small as compared to the increase in risk conferred by the genetic make-up. Other studies have reported no further increase in risk. Our policy is to prescribe HRT to those women with a relevant family history after appropriate counselling. These women must be made aware of their increase in risk and should be offered increased surveillance whether they take HRT or not.

8.40 Do progestogens have an effect upon the risk of breast cancer?

Some years ago it was suggested that progestogens might have a protective effect against breast cancer, and it was advocated that they be added to oestrogens, even in hysterectomized women, for this purpose. However, the majority of studies which have reported a protective effect of combined therapies against breast cancer have been criticized because of small numbers, inclusion bias or failure to control adequately for factors known to influence the risk of breast cancer.

Progestogens exert antimitotic effects upon the endometrium (see Question 6.35). These effects have been extrapolated to breast tissue but, again, it is doubtful whether such an extrapolation is valid. We have already referred (Question 8.27) to evidence that progestogens increase mitosis in breast epithelial tissue. Thus, at this time, there is scant epidemiological and biochemical evidence to support the view that progestogens will protect against breast cancer. Indeed, there is some epidemiological evidence, from very small numbers of women, that the addition of a progestogen may actually increase breast cancer risk.

Because of a lack of evidence supporting a protective effect and because of their potentially undesirable psychological and metabolic side-effects, we do not prescribe progestogens in addition to the oestrogen in hysterectomized women.

8.41 What should I tell a patient about her possible risk of breast cancer?

For many women the fear of breast cancer is the main reason for not taking HRT. Patients need to be informed of the possible risks so that they can make an informed decision. The majority of the better-designed epidemiological studies report no substantial increase in risk with 5 years' use of HRT. It is possible that there is an increase in risk with 10 or more years of HRT, but this remains controversial and some long-term studies report no increase in risk. Regrettably, there is no reliable guide as to which particular sub-group of women is most likely to develop breast cancer.

The factors which will determine the optimal duration of therapy in an individual patient are fully discussed in Chapter 10. It is always important to try to maximize potential benefits and minimize risks. Based upon the currently available evidence, 5 years' use of HRT will achieve skeletal and arterial benefits without compromising breast tissue significantly.

8.42 Is there evidence that the incidence of other cancers is increased with HRT?

No. Epidemiological studies have not shown an association between HRT and some of the other more common cancers such as carcinoma of the colon. The relationship between HRT and malignant melanoma has been discussed earlier in Question 8.24.

8.43 Are there any other established risks of HRT?

The increased incidence of gallstones, the potential for enlargement of fibroids and the reactivation of endometriosis have already been discussed in this chapter. However, these may be considered an aggravation of an existing condition rather than the development of a new disease process.

A recent UK epidemiological study did identify an increased rate of suicide amongst HRT users. This would seem to be an unlikely complication of a treatment that generally improves a woman's sense of wellbeing and therefore it requires further comment. Seven of the 11 patients who committed suicide in this study had a history of psychiatric illness and it may be that these women were prescribed HRT when more specific psychiatric therapy would have been more appropriate. This emphasizes that HRT should not be considered as a panacea for all the ills of middle age, and that severe depression may develop independently of the menopause and ovarian failure. Such depression will not respond to HRT.

8.44 So is HRT safe?

Yes. Given the caveats mentioned earlier in this chapter and concern regarding the possible increased risk of breast cancer with long-term use. In percentage terms, any increase in risk of breast cancer with prolonged use of HRT (if one occurs) is small when compared with the protective effect of HRT upon arterial disease risk. Additionally, far more women die from coronary artery and cerebrovascular disease than from breast cancer (see Question 1.6 and Figure 1.4).

8.45 What is the benefit/risk ratio for HRT?

Given the prevalence of arterial disease and the 40–50% reduction in incidence with HRT, this feature will dominate any such equation. Several epidemiological studies of 'all cause' mortality in HRT-users are underway. Data from the UK study funded by the Medical Research Council are illustrated in Table 8.8. This shows the mortality for HRT-users, compared to non-users, for different causes of death after an average of slightly more than 5 years of HRT exposure. Because this is a UK-based study the patients were taking a wide range of preparations and many (43%) were on oestrogen/progestogen combinations. Several points are noteworthy:

1. The mortality from breast cancer was reduced although the actual incidence of breast cancer was increased by about 60% (data not shown). This reduction in mortality may reflect increased surveillance of patients taking HRT and thus an increased detection of this disease at an early stage. However, other studies have also reported that mortality from breast cancer in HRT-users is reduced, and it is possible that HRT-associated tumours may carry a more favourable prognosis.

2. There were no fatalities from endometrial cancer, although 14 cases were observed (data not shown). On review, 11 were found to have occurred in patients who had taken oestrogen/progestogen therapy. However, in all but one case the progestogen was prescribed either at inadequate daily dose or for an insufficient duration each month for endometrial protection.

3. Slightly more cases of ovarian cancer were observed than expected but, on pathological review, two were found to be secondary deposits from colon cancer.

Table 8.8 Mortality by cause of death

Cause of death	Number of observed deaths	Number of expected deaths	Observed/ expected
Breast cancer	12	21.9	0.55
Endometrial cancer	0	2.06	–
Ovarian cancer	8	7.13	1.12
Ischaemic heart disease	20	42.04	0.48
Cerebrovascular accident	14	21.64	0.65
Suicide	11	4.34	2.53
All causes	124	212.5	0.58

(From Hunt K, Vessey M, McPherson K, Coleman M 1987 British Journal of Obstetrics and Gynaecology 94, 620–635. Reproduced with permission.)

4. The data on cardiovascular disease are particularly important as these are early data on a group of patients of whom slightly less than half were taking oestrogen/progestogen combinations. Overall, these results show a 50% reduction in incidence, which is very similar to that seen in users of oestrogen-only therapy (see Question 4.32). This suggests that the fear that progestogen addition negates the cardio-protective effects of oestrogens is overstated. More data on the arterial effects of combined therapies are urgently required.

5. The reduction in risk of stroke (relative risk 0.65) is similar to that observed in patients taking unopposed oestrogens.

6. The surprising increase in incidence of suicide has already been commented upon earlier in this Chapter.

The net reduction in mortality in the HRT-users is over 40%. However, long-term studies are awaited to help determine the optimal duration of therapy.

9. Assessment, monitoring and problems on treatment

Patients seeking medical advice are either symptomatic or asymptomatic but, in general, the basic assessment is the same in the two groups. For each patient, it should be determined that an indication for HRT is present and that no absolute contraindications to oestrogen therapy exist. One of the primary objectives of the consultation is to help the patient weigh the relative merits and disadvantages of taking HRT, taking into account her past, present and future health needs. Patients need to be allowed time to make an informed decision.

9.1 What are the general principles of assessment?

Standard techniques are used; observation, history taking, physical examination and investigations followed by interpretation of the information obtained.

9.2 Why do patients seek advice regarding menopausal problems?

Patients seek advice for four major reasons: because they undoubtedly have troublesome oestrogen-deficiency symptoms (see Table 3.1); because they have symptoms that they believe are due to oestrogen deficiency; because they have concerns (usually from personal experience of a relative) regarding later osteoporosis or arterial disease, and finally because they have heard about HRT and want more information.

9.3 Where do women obtain information about the menopause and HRT?

From the outset, some women seek advice from their general practitioner or other member of the primary health care team. However, a recent study has shown that more women obtain information about the menopause and HRT from the mass media or a friend rather than from a health care professional. This study also reported that more than 20% of patients had exerted pressure on their general practitioner to obtain more information about HRT. Publicity in the mass media may influence the demand for information and for therapy; importantly, it may also affect a woman's expectations and perceptions of treatment.

9.4 Should GPs initiate a discussion of the problems of the climacteric with all their female patients approaching the menopause?

We believe so. We see no good reason why all women should not have access to information about the menopause. It is important that this be accurate and presented impartially. The members of the primary health care team seem best placed to do this, whether directly through counselling services themselves or indirectly by supplying reading and other information material. All women will experience the climacteric and while not all will suffer severe symptoms, all of them are potentially at risk from the long-term sequelae of oestrogen deficiency. If men routinely experienced gonadal failure in middle life we would expect a similar and perfectly reasonable demand for information from them.

A discussion of menopause-related issues will not necessarily result in a prescription for HRT; it does, however, provide an opportunity for general health education and screening which may be as, if not more, important. There is some evidence that it is those who are better off financially and better educated who attend menopause clinics and request HRT. However, because all women should be involved with general health education and screening, all women in the relevant age group (40–60 years) should be invited to attend an appropriate consultation (Well Woman Clinic or Health Promotion Clinic). Response rates to such invitations are always less than 100% and therefore the primary health care team should consider a 'catch-all' approach with opportunistic case finding. These activities will identify some women suffering symptoms for which they thought no treatment was available, as well as some women who were unaware of their personal risks of osteoporosis or heart disease.

9.5 Should GPs regard some women as high risk and in particular need of advice?

If one group is going to be selected then it should be those women who have undergone premature menopause. The earlier the age at menopause the greater the risk of both osteoporosis and heart disease. Identical comments apply to women experiencing prolonged periods of amenorrhoea and hypo-oestrogenism during the reproductive era (see Question 5.13).

9.6 How can such women be identified?

Premature menopause may be either spontaneous, surgically induced, or result from therapies for life-threatening conditions such as leukaemia. Women falling into the two latter categories may be identified from the medical records. This is a time-consuming exercise even if summary cards are available in each patient's case-notes. Computerised record systems, however, make this task relatively simple. An alternative approach is for every member of the primary health care team to be aware of the problems that the menopause may bring and in particular to remember that the premature menopause carries a special risk.

HISTORY TAKING

9.7 How should GP's approach the first consultation?

Initially, the patient's motive for seeking advice should be identified. The majority of patients will present with climacteric symptoms, and a minority will be asymptomatic.

It is not for us to dictate the degree of detail of the history. This will depend, in part, upon whether the consultation is being conducted with a typical symptomatic woman or as part of a general health screen. The importance of asking specific questions relating to symptoms due to oestrogen deficiency, if there is any doubt about the diagnosis, has already been stressed (see Question 5.2). Because the use of oestrogens will be influenced by many previous medical conditions (jaundice, thrombosis, endometrial hyperplasia, endometriosis, fibroids, breast lumps, etc.), and because the risks of osteoporosis and arterial disease are affected not only by the individual patient's lifestyle but also by her family history, a comprehensive history will be long and detailed. Such a history (which will most probably make most family practitioners throw up their hands in despair!) is illustrated in Appendix 1.

9.8 What methods can be adopted to hasten history taking since available time may be limited?

Some health care professionals find it helpful to draw up a record card including a check list to cover the major points of the history. We believe that the value of a practice nurse in assisting with history taking is greatly underestimated.

If a regular Well Woman/Menopause Clinic is in operation the patient can be requested to complete a questionnaire outlining the basic medical history and perhaps a symptom rating scale. Some family practitioners may wish to do preliminary work by reviewing the patient's current medical record and entering details on the menopause clinic card.

9.9 Will all patients wish to take HRT?

No. Some patients do not wish to take hormones and some who initially request HRT may change their mind after an assessment of the relative benefits and disadvantages of treatment.

EXAMINATION

9.10 What is required in the pre-HRT screen?

A general physical examination should be performed, including measurements of height, weight and blood pressure. The value of routine urinalysis in a pre-HRT screen (as compared to a general health screen) has not been determined. Breast and pelvic examinations (with cervical smear if appropriate) should be performed, with any abnormalities so discovered being investigated in the usual way.

Again, a practice nurse can provide considerable assistance.

9.11 What is the purpose of the pelvic examination?

The state of the vulval and vaginal epithelium should be assessed together with any degree of prolapse. The cervix should be inspected and a cervical smear taken (if indicated). Uterine size should be determined and any adnexal masses must be noted.

Current advice is that the frequency of cervical smears is not changed by the prescription of HRT.

INVESTIGATIONS

9.12 What investigations are routinely required?

No additional investigations are required in most women. In particular, hormone profiles are usually unnecessary.

9.13 When are additional investigations required?

The need for these is influenced by points in the history and abnormal clinical findings.

1. There may be symptoms and signs suggestive of disorders such as anaemia or thyroid disease, and therefore a full blood count or thyroid function tests will be required.

2. A patient with a relevant past history of thrombo-embolism (see Question 8.7) may require a full fibrinolysis/coagulation profile, e.g. KCCT, antithrombin III, and protein S and C levels (see Question 8.8).

3. If a breast lump or pelvic mass is detected then this will require appropriate management.

4. A patient with a relevant past history of a benign breast lump and/or a strong relevant family history of breast cancer should be considered for a screening mammography whether HRT is or is not taken (see Questions 8.38 and 8.39).

5. Very occasionally, serum FSH measurements may be useful, e.g. (a) to confirm premature menopause (see Question 5.7); (b) to confirm ovarian failure following previous hysterectomy (see Questions 5.3 and 5.4); and (c) where the diagnosis is uncertain (see Question 9.16).

9.14 Should all women have a mammogram before commencing HRT?

As discussed in Question 8.35 there is scant evidence that the currently prescribed HRT formulations, when administered for durations up to 5 years, increase breast cancer risk significantly.

Our policy is as follows. We advise all women aged 50 years and over who have not undergone mammography in the previous 3 years to consider having one performed. This policy follows the recommendation of the Forrest Report and is not influenced by use of HRT. As the National Breast Cancer Screening Service enlarges, more facilities will become available nationwide.

Certain patients must be considered at high risk for breast cancer, whether they take HRT or not. These include women with a first degree relative who developed this disease premenopausally, and women with a personal history of 'benign' breast disease especially those with histologically proven lobular and/or ductal hyperplasia; some authorities would also include epitheliosis with atypia. Surveillance of these women is much more influenced by the family or personal history than by use of HRT. The optimal frequency of mammograms in this group is not clear because surgical opinions appear divided (annually, every second year); identical comments apply to the age at which mammography is first offered, be this 40 or 45 years.

There are no data to support or refute the value of the routine use of mammography in women starting HRT under age 50 years.

9.15 Do women need dilatation and curettage (D&C) or endometrial sampling prior to HRT?

No. Extensive research has shown that this is unnecessary in non-hysterectomized women provided that an adequate course of progestogen is prescribed together with the oestrogen.

It has been shown that pre-malignant endometrial pathology can exist, pre-HRT, in 1–2% of postmenopausal women who have not bled for 12 months. In the majority of cases (over 95%) the endometrial abnormality is reversed by combined oestrogen/progestogen therapy. The small minority of women in whom the abnormality does not revert to normal usually experience abnormal uterine bleeding during the first 3–4 months of HRT. An endometrial biopsy is then indicated and the abnormality is thereby unmasked.

However, it must be remembered that unopposed oestrogens given to patients with pre-existing hyperplasia can lead to the rapid development of endometrial carcinoma (see Question 8.32). If unopposed oestrogens are to be prescribed to non-hysterectomized, postmenopausal women it is probably advisable to perform a pre-treatment endometrial biopsy. Unopposed oestrogen supplements can be prescribed to premenopausal women with regular cycles provided that endogenous progesterone production is adequate for endometrial protection (see Question 5.18).

9.16 Are hormone profiles necessary prior to HRT?

Rarely. In most patients the diagnosis is straightforward because the symptoms are typical in nature and closely associated with oligomenorrhoea or amenorrhoea. It must be remembered that plasma gonadotrophin (FSH and LH) and oestrogen concentrations fluctuate widely during the climacteric and, therefore, biochemical investigations are of little value in diagnosis and symptoms are always the best guide. In addition, hormone profiles are of little guide to the eventual severity or duration of symptoms, or to their response to therapy.

However, there are some exceptions. For example, at least two hormone profiles will be necessary to diagnose spontaneous premature menopause. Secondly, investigations may be indicated to confirm ovarian failure after hysterectomy (see Question 5.3) and will be required to diagnose premature ovarian failure (see Question 5.7). Thirdly, endocrine investigations may be helpful where the diagnosis is uncertain. For example, when symptoms are non-specific, menstruation is fairly regular and vasomotor problems are absent. Here a raised FSH may be indicative of the early climacteric but again it is stressed that such investigations are not always reliable and a therapeutic trial of HRT may be the best course of action.

9.17 Should all women have a pelvic ultrasound examination prior to HRT?

No. This is not necessary in the absence of a clinical abnormality.

The effects of HRT upon the risk of ovarian cancer have been discussed in Question 8.31.

Evidence is emerging that a strong family history is an important predictor for ovarian cancer. Therefore, pelvic ultrasonography may be indicated in women with a family history of this disease whether they take HRT or not. However, further research is required in this area.

9.18 Should all women have a lipid screen prior to HRT?

The indications for lipid screening are unaffected by a patient's request for HRT. Therefore, the family practitioner should apply his or her usual criteria such as a strong family history of arterial disease (especially in relatives developing arterial disease under age 60 years), hypertension, cigarette smoking, obesity, diabetes, xanthelasma, etc.

9.19 Should all women have a bone density assessment prior to HRT?

This is not possible as resources are very scarce. Where facilities are available a bone densitometry scan is of particular value for women who, in the absence of climacteric symptoms, would take HRT if they were shown to be at risk of later osteoporosis. Plain X-rays are of no value as a screening tool because 20–25% of bone mass has to be lost before radiological change is apparent. It has been suggested that certain biochemical markers could be used as a screening tool. However, the value of such tests is not yet proven in multi-centre studies. Screening for osteoporosis is discussed in Question 5.27.

COUNSELLING THE PATIENT

9.20 What factors should be borne in mind when counselling the patient?

More women identify a friend or the mass media as their first source of information about the menopause, osteoporosis and HRT than the health care professional. While some of this information will be accurate, almost inevitably some sources are less well informed. In addition, information can be misunderstood or misinterpreted. Patients turn to their family doctor, nurse or health visitor for reliable informed advice. Therefore, during history taking it is important to establish how much the patient already knows, and to be prepared to deal with her queries, dispel any myths, correct all inaccuracies and give an overall balanced view.

Finally, it should not be forgotten that patients may require contraceptive advice. It is important to inform patients that the oestrogen doses commonly prescribed in HRT are not contraceptive. See Chapter 12.

9.21 How much information do patients usually require?

Discussion should cover the short and long-term consequences of the menopause, the likely benefits and possible risks of HRT, the types of HRT available, the disadvantages of therapy (e.g. regular periods, side-effects), the surveillance needed before and while on therapy, and finally the proposed duration of treatment. Discussions can, of course, take place over a series of visits. A considerable amount of patient education literature in the form of leaflets, books, audio cassettes, etc. are now available (see page 224). Most women value the opportunity to discuss the menopause and HRT with a professional. While explanation and reassurance may be all that is required, there is an opportunity to give general health education advice (regarding diet, exercise, smoking, alcohol etc.) and to provide screening services (e.g. blood pressure, breast examination, cervical smear, etc.).

9.22 What are the most common anxieties about HRT among patients?

Most anxieties relate to aspects of HRT safety and its side-effects, or to the fear of 'interfering with nature'.

Perhaps the most common fear is that HRT causes cancer, in particular, breast cancer. Some women may also fear heart attacks and strokes, and some of these worries may have been generated by confusion between HRT and the oral contraceptive pill. These issues require full discussion with the patient in the light of recent research. The oral contraceptive pill and HRT appear to have markedly different effects upon arterial disease risk (see Question 4.32).

Some patients have a fear of HRT because it involves the use of hormones which they regard as 'dangerous drugs'. The plasma oestradiol levels achieved with oral and transdermal therapies are within the premenopausal, mid-proliferative phase range; those achieved with implants can be higher (see Questions 6.5 and 6.16) but, clearly, if oestrogens were significantly damaging to the health then most women would not survive to reach menopause. It should be emphasised that HRT uses natural oestrogen in relatively small doses (see Chapter 6).

While no-one would argue that the menopause is not a natural event patients should be reassured that HRT is not given for frivolous reasons. It is not an elixir of youth and although many women find that their quality of life is improved the ageing process continues unabated.

9.23 In what ways do women interpret their symptoms?

There is enormous variability. Some women recognise their symptoms as being due to ovarian failure. Others, however, describe quite typical climacteric symptoms yet do not recognize them as such, believing instead that they have a psychological, psychiatric or even serious physical aetiology such as undiagnosed cancer, heart disease or arthritis. Yet other women, who clearly do not have oestrogen-deficiency symptoms, may attribute all their ills 'to the menopause' – even though they may have experienced problems for 20 years prior to menopause. The latter group can be difficult to reason with and they may be reluctant to consider any alternative explanation other than menopause.

9.24 How should we help the patient come to a decision about her need for HRT?

By presenting accurate information about the benefits and risks in a balanced, impartial manner. Most patients can then make an informed decision. For those who find it difficult to do this even when fully informed a trial of therapy can be offered (see Question 5.15). Because some patients are very concerned about possible side-effects, it is important to emphasize that treatment can be stopped at any time.

9.25 What advice should be given to a patient on starting HRT?

The side-effects that occur on starting HRT have been discussed in Questions 7.2 and 7.3. These include nausea, breast tenderness and leg cramps but they usually resolve spontaneously within the first few weeks.

Maximal compliance will be achieved if the patient feels confident about and comfortable with therapy. In our experience, one of the simplest ways of achieving these aims is to show the patient the HRT preparation that she will use. This applies to implants (demonstrated prior to insertion) as well as to pills and patches. In patients about to start combined oestrogen/progestogen regimens, the progestogen phase of treatment should be clearly defined and the time when the withdrawal bleed will occur must be indicated. We issue charts to the patient to assist this educational process. Sample charts for oral oestrogens and transdermal oestrogens are shown in Figures 9.1 and 9.2: with both, the progestogen is given orally. Patients are requested to complete the chart during the oestrogen and progestogen treatment phases (to serve as a check on compliance), and to record all vaginal bleeding. Breakthrough bleeding can then be differentiated from progestogen-associated or withdrawal bleeding. The former is not uncommon at the start of therapy but seldom lasts more than a couple of days, is usually light and has resolved by the end of the second treatment cycle. It resembles the breakthrough bleeding commonly seen in younger women starting the oral contraceptive pill.

By monitoring the pattern of withdrawal bleeding, the endometrial status may be assessed and the need for biopsy reduced if not obviated (see Question 9.30). All this may take from as short as 2 minutes to as long as 10 minutes, and our clinic sisters perform this important instruction session. It cannot be emphasized strongly enough that this time will reduce patient concerns and, most importantly, will minimize the number of phone calls and follow-up visits from patients anxious, in particular, about bleeding. It is time well spent.

Patients should be encouraged to perform regular breast self-examination, and to change their lifestyle and thereby reduce risk factors for osteoporosis and arterial disease if these are present.

The need for regular surveillance should be explained. The first follow-up visit is usually after 3 months; thereafter, alternate visits could be undertaken by an experienced practice nurse (see Question 9.28).

Finally, patients should be given details of whom to contact should they need advice. We appreciate that many primary health care physicians may not have a practice nurse and will respond to queries in their usual manner. However, the availability of an experienced practice nurse, even for 2 hours each week for telephone counselling, can be invaluable.

		PATIENT DIARY
Date recordings on this sheet started: └─┴─┴─┘ day / month / year		

Tablet taken: Please mark with a **cross** on the appropriate line those days when you take a tablet

Bleeding: Please mark with a **cross** (on the appropriate line indicating the strength) the day(s) you experience vaginal bleeding

Day of this treatment cycle:		1	2	3	4	5	6	7	8	9	10	11	12	13	14	15	16	17	18	19	20	21	22	23	24	25	26	27	28
Day of week:																													
Oestrogen tablet																													
Progestogen tablet																													
Bleeding:	Spotting																												
	Slight																												
	Medium																												
	Strong																												

Occurrence of any symptoms?

If yes: What? When?
Please note here any details
and indicate the *day of treatment*
cycle the symptom occurred
(write in block capitals only)

Fig. 9.1 Sample bleeding chart for patients taking oral oestrogens and oral progestogens.

9.26 What are the common questions that patients ask?

At the visit when HRT is prescribed, patients often ask about the risks of cancer, thrombosis, unwanted hair growth, weight gain etc., with HRT. These are fully discussed elsewhere in this book.

MONITORING

9.27 What is the procedure at the first follow-up visit?

This usually takes place towards the end of a 3-month course of HRT because this is most often the time needed to achieve maximum benefits in relieving vasomotor symptoms (see Question 5.15 and Fig. 5.4).

Enquiry should be made as to whether symptoms are well controlled, and whether or not side-effects have occurred and whether they are still present. In non-hysterectomized women, enquiry should be made as to whether withdrawal bleeding has or has not occurred. As discussed in Question 6.29, overall approximately 85% of women taking conventional, combined

| Date recordings on this sheet started: ⌴⌴⌴ day / month / year | **PATIENT DIARY** |

Treatment: Please mark with a **cross** on the appropriate line those days when you apply a new patch

Bleeding: Please mark with a **cross** (on the appropriate line indicating the strength) the day(s) you experience vaginal bleeding

Day of this treatment cycle:	1	2	3	4	5	6	7	8	9	10	11	12	13	14	15	16	17	18	19	20	21	22	23	24	25	26	27	28
Day of week:																												
Oestrogen patch																												
Progestogen tablet																												
Bleeding: Spotting																												
Slight																												
Medium																												
Strong																												

Occurrence of any **symptoms?**

If yes: What?   When?
*Please note here any details
and indicate the <u>day of treatment
cycle</u> the symptom occurred
(write in block capitals only)*

Fig. 9.2 Sample bleeding chart for patients taking transdermal oestrogens and oral progestogens.

oestrogen/progestogen regimens (in which the oestrogen is given for 21 or 28 days, and the progestogen is added for 7–12 days each cycle) will experience the re-establishment of withdrawal bleeding. This will depend upon the oestrogen dose. If this has occurred, the day of onset of the bleeding, the duration and the amount of flow should be assessed. The 'average' woman will bleed for approximately 4–8 days and the flow should resemble that of a 'normal' period experienced during the reproductive era. Use of bleeding charts (Figs 9.1 and 9.2) enables the physician to obtain this information easily. Abnormal bleeding is discussed further below. Traditionally, the weight and blood pressure are recorded although the value of these measurements is debatable.

Strategies to overcome specific problems due either to therapy failing to control symptoms adequately, or because it has caused unacceptable side-effects are discussed later in this chapter.

Health education advice (regular breast self-examination; diet; exercise; stress management; reduction in tobacco and alcohol consumption) should be reinforced. A further follow-up visit is arranged, usually for six months time. Thereafter, we see patients every 12–18 months.

9.28 What tests are required during therapy and how frequently should they be performed?

It is standard practice to record the weight and blood pressure at each visit. However, placebo-controlled studies have failed to demonstrate a weight gain with oral oestrogen therapy of more than 2–3 lb. Large scale studies of oral therapy indicate that a significant rise in blood pressure occurs in only 1–2% of women, and one report has suggested that, long term, the blood pressure is most likely to rise significantly only in those women who gain weight excessively (see Question 7.3). Because breast cancer is the commonest hormone-dependent cancer, we believe it sensible to perform breast examinations every 12–18 months. In accord with the recommendations of the Forrest Report, we advise women aged 50–64 years to undergo mammography every 3 years – not because they are on HRT but because of their age. Many specialists would recommend that certain women in high risk groups undergo mammography every 1–2 years, e.g. women with a strong, relevant family history of breast cancer or previous relevant surgically confirmed benign breast disease (see Questions 8.34, 8.36, 8.38 and 9.14).

Cervical smears should be performed regularly every 3–5 years as per standard protocols. A pelvic examination should be performed at this time. It is doubtful whether more frequent pelvic examinations are of any benefit.

9.29 What additional tests may be performed?

No additional tests are required for most women. However, in some cases further investigations may be indicated. For example, a follow-up measurement of serum cholesterol may help to motivate hypercholesterolaemic patients on low cholesterol diets.

Women with a history of endometriosis or fibroids should receive careful supervision. This will usually involve regular clinical pelvic examinations (perhaps every 6–12 months) and often pelvic ultrasound examination if symptoms and/or signs of growth of fibroids or reactivation of endometiotic disease occur.

9.30 Are regular D&Cs or endometrial sampling needed in women receiving combined oestrogen/progestogen regimens?

The overwhelming majority of women will be receiving a sequential combined oestrogen/progestogen regimen in which the oestrogen is administered for 21 or 28 days and the progestogen is added for 12–13 days of each cycle (see Question 6.39). Approximately 85% of women will have withdrawal bleeding with this type of regimen. Our current understanding is that regular endometrial sampling is not required if the following criteria are fulfilled:

1. The withdrawal bleeding is not heavier than the 'normal' period experienced during the reproductive era;

2. The withdrawal bleed lasts for a similar duration to the 'normal' period experienced during the reproductive era (in most women this is 4–8 days), and

3. The withdrawal bleeding starts with orally administered oestrogens on the 10th/11th day of progestogen addition or later, and with transdermal oestrogens on the 8th/9th day of oral progestogen addition or later.

There is a correlation between the day of onset of bleeding and the endometrial status. The data for oral oestrogens are shown in Figure 9.3. The mean day of onset of bleeding (over a 3-month period) was calculated and correlated with the endometrial histology. The vertical axis shows the days of progestogen addition (with day 12 being the last day). Bleeding starting on day 11 or later was associated with progestational effects within the endometrium.

Similar data have been published for transdermal oestrogens. For reasons that are incompletely understood, the bleeding may start earlier with transdermal oestrogen therapy (on day 8 or day 9 of oral progestogen addition), yet progestational activity within the endometrium is still observed.

Continuous/combined oestrogen/progestogen therapies (in which both the oestrogen and progestogen are administered every day, continuously) have been advocated by some authorities. The aim has been to induce amenorrhoea but our experience has been disappointing. Chronic, irregular bleeding is common and results in many women discontinuing treatment. As yet, there are no long-term endometrial, safety data on continuous/combined oestrogen/progestogen regimens. Additionally, there are no clear guidelines as to the frequency of endometrial sampling. We believe that continuous/combined treatments should be restricted to research units until more data become available.

If women who have not had a hysterectomy receive unopposed oestrogen therapy, endometrial samples are required regularly (at least once per year), irrespective of the presence or absence of bleeding and whether it is regular. There are at least two reports that unopposed oestrogens increase the risk of endometrial cancer for many years after such therapy is withdrawn, and therefore unopposed oestrogens appear to have a prolonged 'carry-over' effect (see Question 8.32). Thus, the decision to prescribe unopposed oestrogens to postmenopausal women should not be taken lightly.

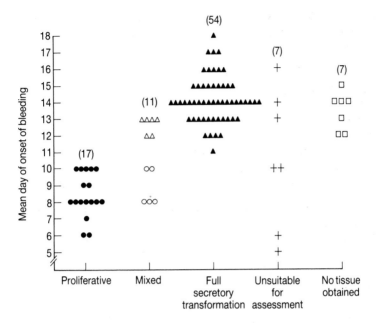

Fig. 9.3 Correlation of endometrial histology versus day of onset of bleeding after addition of the progestogen. Number of samples shown in parentheses. (From Padwick M L, Pryse-Davies J, Whitehead M I 1986 New England Journal of Medicine 315: 930–934. Reproduced with permission.)

PROBLEMS ON TREATMENT

9.31 What are the most common problems on treatment?

These usually fall into one or more of three categories:

1. failure to control symptoms adequately;
2. abnormal bleeding, and
3. side-effects of treatment.

The latter are considered in Chapter 7.

9.32 What may cause inadequate symptom relief?

The failure of HRT to control a patient's symptoms may be due to one or more of the following:

1. an inadequate dose of oestrogen;
2. inadequate absorption and/or poor compliance;
3. drug interactions;

4. an inadequate duration of therapy;
5. symptoms not due to oestrogen deficiency, and
6. unrealistic expectations.

9.33 What are the average dosages required?

The usual starting doses for the relief of typical vasomotor symptoms are shown in Table 9.1. By moderate symptoms we mean up to six flushes per day and up to two sweats each night; severe symptoms are more frequent vasomotor disturbances. Some relief of symptoms is usually experienced within 2–3 weeks but maximal benefits may not be achieved for 3 months. Therefore, the oestrogen dose should not be increased too soon after HRT has been commenced; if it is, then symptoms of oestrogen overdosage (breast tenderness, bloatedness) may result.

9.34 How may the route of administration be important?

To achieve the desired effect, sufficient oestrogen must reach the target tissues. Clearly, this will not be achieved if compliance has been poor. However, the route of administration may also affect absorption. Some women may not absorb oral oestrogen adequately from the bowel and we have seen this problem more frequently in women who have undergone surgical resection for small bowel disease (see Question 5.22). In theory, poor absorption might occur with transdermal application but this does not appear to be a problem in practice. The subcutaneous route has the advantage that compliance is guaranteed and poor absorption, in our experience, occurs rarely only when the implant site becomes infected (see Question 7.6). The oestrogen doses usually administered vaginally are so small that they will only relieve mild vasomotor symptoms.

If symptoms are not controlled adequately despite the use of the maximal oral dose a change to one of the non-oral routes is well worthwhile.

9.35 What drugs may reduce oestrogen benefits?

With all routes of administration, various drugs may interfere with oestrogen metabolism and thereby reduce efficacy. Antibiotics can cause intestinal 'hurry', and change the bowel flora; entero-hepatic recycling (the second-pass effect: see Question 6.6) may be disturbed and the overall oestrogenic stimulation is thereby reduced. This may be why antibiotics appear to be a potent cause of breakthrough bleeding in women taking HRT. Identical comments apply to episodes of diarrhoea. Other drugs may increase the activity of the liver enzymes responsible for oestrogen

Table 9.1 Recommended doses of oestrogen for relief of vasomotor symptoms

Preparation	Vasomotor symptoms		
	Mild	Moderate	Severe
Oral			
conjugated equine oestrogens (Premarin® – Wyeth-Ayerst)	0.625 mg	0.625 mg	1.25 mg
piperazine oestrone sulphate (Harmogen® – Abbott)	0.75 mg	1.5 mg	3 mg
oestradiol valerate (Progynova® – Schering)	1 mg	2 mg	2–4 mg
Non-oral			
transdermal oestradiol (Estraderm® – Ciba-Geigy)	25 μg	50 μg	100 μg
subcutaneous oestradiol (implant – Organon)	25–50 mg	50 mg	50–100 mg

metabolism and in so doing accelerate oestrogen clearance; the most well recognized are the barbiturates phenytoin and carbamazepine.

9.36 How may the duration of therapy be important?

Symptom relief may be inadequate if oestrogen is prescribed cyclically rather than continuously. In the past, oestrogens were given for 21 out of every 28 days and some preparations still include a treatment-free week. In our experience, this practice commonly results in the return of symptoms during the oestrogen-free week in patients with frequent and severe vasomotor disturbances. The ovary continues to produce oestradiol throughout the ovulatory cycle (small doses are produced during menstruation), and a treatment-free week from oestrogen is unphysiological.

9.37 What else may explain the failure of HRT to relieve symptoms?

If an adequate dose of HRT administered for an appropriate duration and via an appropriate route fails to relieve symptoms then it is very probable that the symptom is not due to oestrogen deficiency. This occurs very, very infrequently with hot flushes but other causes must then be considered. These include thyroid disease, phaeochromocytoma and carcinoid syndrome. We have seen only one patient with one of these conditions during the last 10 years.

However, the failure of response of other symptoms such as anxiety, depression, lethargy, aching joints and stress incontinence is more frequent because these symptoms can be due to factors other than oestrogen deficiency. Other causes and treatments should then be pursued.

Perhaps one of the most difficult areas is a complaint of loss of libido which may be multi-factorial in origin. Some patients undoubtedly derive considerable benefit from HRT whilst others find it less helpful or of minimal benefit (see Question 4.10).

9.38 What other factors may play a role?

Some patients complain that they have not derived symptomatic benefits from HRT. Often these are the women who hold unrealistic expectations of therapy. This problem may be fuelled by the popular press and relate to cosmetic changes or psychological aspects of the menopause. This serves to emphasize the importance of counselling patients adequately before initiating HRT.

It is important to remember that asymptomatic women taking HRT as prophylactic treatment often derive no physical or psychological benefits.

9.39 What sort of problems may occur with vaginal bleeding?

The criteria for a normal withdrawal bleed were defined earlier in this chapter (see Question 9.30). The withdrawal bleeding may be abnormal because although it occurs at the appropriate time in the cycle it is too heavy, lasts too long or is associated with significant pain. Alternatively, bleeding may occur during the cycle unrelated to the phase of progestogen addition; this is called breakthrough bleeding.

9.40 How should breakthrough bleeding be investigated?

Although breakthrough bleeding is abnormal it is, perhaps surprisingly, seldom due to intrauterine pathology in our experience. The most important non-invasive investigation is an adequate history because breakthrough bleeding commonly results from causes which are not sinister. These include:

1. Failure of compliance

This is most probably the commonest cause of breakthrough bleeding. Missing one or two oestrogen or progestogen tablets can result in breakthrough bleeding. Forgetting to change a patch at the appropriate time gives an identical result. We have observed a higher incidence of breakthrough bleeding in patients on transdermal therapy during the months of July and August, and this most probably represents interruption to the normal routine during the summer holiday.

2. *Drug interactions*

Those drugs interfering with oestrogen metabolism were discussed in Question 9.35. Antibiotics are a common cause of breakthrough bleeding with both oral and transdermal oestrogen therapies; so are episodes of diarrhoea. For obvious reasons, vomiting will reduce oral oestrogen and progestogen availability and may result in breakthrough bleeding.

3. *A surge of spontaneous ovarian activity?*

This was discussed in Question 5.19. The typical history is of bleeding, often described as being like a normal period, preceded by typical prodromal symptoms (irritability, breast tenderness, etc.). It is much more common in peri- as compared to postmenopausal women taking HRT.

4. *Stress, especially if it includes long-distance travel*

We have frequently observed this phenomenon but the mechanism of action is quite unknown, unless it is due to poor compliance.

We do not routinely submit patients to invasive investigation because of one episode of breakthrough bleeding which can be explained by one of the above factors.

Two or more episodes of breakthrough bleeding demand appropriate investigation, i.e. D&C or endometrial biopsy. Even then, sinister intrauterine pathology is seldom found but polyps, endometrial hyperplasia and carcinoma must be excluded in patients with recurrent breakthrough bleeding.

9.41 How should the problems of heavy and/or prolonged and/or painful withdrawal bleeding be investigated and managed?

Withdrawal bleeding occurring at the appropriate time during the cycle which is abnormal because it is excessively heavy, lasts too long or is associated with excessive pain may result from a number of causes. The commonest are:

1. *Constitutional*

Women who had heavy, prolonged, painful periods during the reproductive era are more likely to experience this pattern if they take HRT. This can be a very difficult problem to overcome. Reducing the oestrogen dose may help, but such dosage reductions may compromise symptomatic benefits and the protective effect on bone conservation may be lost (see Question 6.27 and Table 6.4).

2. Associated with unopposed oestrogen stimulation

In untreated women, the peri- and postmenopausal ovary may continue to produce small amounts of oestradiol which, over a period of time, can result in significant endometrial stimulation. After starting HRT, withdrawal of the progestogen at the end of the first treatment month with combined HRT will result in sloughing of this excess endometrial tissue. The result is a heavy and prolonged withdrawal bleed. *All patients should be warned that the first one or two withdrawal bleeds may be heavier and last longer than those experienced subsequently.* Obviously, this problem resolves spontaneously, usually by the third treatment month.

3. Fibroids

These cause menorrhagia. Fibroids are oestrogen-dependent and can enlarge during HRT. They may achieve considerable size and we have seen patients with fibroids as large as a 16–18-week pregnancy.

The patient with fibroids causing significant menorrhagia has two choices; to stop HRT or to consider surgery (almost certainly hysterectomy). In our experience, patients with moderate to severe climacteric symptoms often choose the latter; women with minimal symptoms are much more likely to stop treatment.

4. Endometrial polyps

These can cause heavy withdrawal bleeding, breakthrough bleeding and also a blood-stained vaginal discharge. They are the only intrauterine pathology which is not reliably detected by outpatient endometrial biopsy and, often, are only diagnosed at D&C. They are seldom malignant, and seldom cause uterine enlargement.

5. Endometrial hyperplasia and carcinoma

Like polyps these, too, can cause heavy withdrawal bleeding, breakthrough bleeding and also a blood-stained vaginal discharge. Unlike polyps, they are reliably diagnosed using out-patient endometrial sampling techniques. Early endometrial carcinoma may not be associated with uterine enlargement.

6. *An inadequate progestogen dose*

The typical presenting features are of withdrawal bleeding which regularly starts early during the phase of progestogen addition, often around day 4–6. For the first 2 or 3 days the bleeding is very light and is often described by the patient as 'spotting' or a brown/black discharge. The subsequent menstrual flow is relatively normal. The presentation closely resembles that not uncommonly seen in women who from their early 40s are approaching the end of the reproductive era and in whom progesterone production may be inadequate – the so-called 'inadequate luteal phase'.

Treatment is aimed at increasing the progestogen dose. This is discussed further in Question 9.42.

7. *Other pelvic pathology*

Significant dysmenorrhoea, especially when associated with deep dyspareunia, raises the suspicion of organic pelvic pathology such as endometriosis. This, like fibroids, is an oestrogen-dependent condition and is considered further in Question 9.45.

9.42 How should abnormal withdrawal bleeding be investigated?

From the above list of possible diagnoses, heavy withdrawal bleeding occurring at the start of treatment should be obvious and usually resolves spontaneously. If it does not then the diagnosis must be reviewed and a biopsy must be considered.

Abnormal bleeding due to an inadequate progestogen dose is best managed by increasing the progestogen dose. This will be straightforward if the patient is taking a combined therapy 'made up' by the physician (see Question 6.40). However, it may be more difficult to achieve if the patient is using a fixed-dose combination regimen produced by one of the drug manufacturers.

With fixed-dose combinations, the progestogen dose can be increased with Prempak-C® (Wyeth-Ayerst), which contains conjugated equine oestrogens and norgestrel as the progestogen, by supplementing with one or two Neogest® (Schering) tablets (each containing 75 μg norgestrel) during the progestogen phase of treatment. An identical strategy holds for Cyclo-Progynova® (Schering) which also contains norgestrel as the progestogen. Trisequens® (Novo-Nordisk) and Estrapak® (Ciba-Geigy) use norethisterone as the progestogen; supplementation can be achieved with one or two Micronor® (Ortho-Cilag) tablets (each containing 0.35 mg norethisterone), again prescribed during the progestogen phase of treatment. If this strategy is ineffective within 3-4 months then the diagnosis must be reviewed and biopsy must be seriously considered.

Intrauterine pathology must also be considered with all of the other suspected causes of abnormal withdrawal bleeding. The long-term management of patients with fibroids has been referred to. Because fibroids may rarely co-exist with polyps and other more sinister endometrial pathologies (hyperplasia and carcinoma) the counsel of perfection in patients with fibroids is to perform endometrial biopsy to exclude these other intrauterine causes.

As indicated previously, pelvic pathology must be suspected in patients with abnormal withdrawal bleeding who also complain of significant dysmenorrhoea and have other symptoms, such as deep dyspareunia. If adnexal swellings (suggestive of ovarian enlargement) are also detected either by clinical examination or by pelvic ultrasound then laparoscopy will almost certainly be required as well as D&C. In our experience, this symptom-complex occurs infrequently and the commonest cause is endometriosis. We believe this condition to be worthy of special consideration (see Question 9.45).

In summary, therefore, all patients with withdrawal bleeding that is significantly heavier than that experienced during the reproductive era; which lasts longer and which has not responded to an increase in progestogen dose (if an inadequate progestogen dose was considered the most likely diagnosis) need to be considered for endometrial biopsy: those in whom adnexal pathology is suspected will almost certainly require laparoscopy as well.

9.43 How should patients who develop endometrial hyperplasia during combined oestrogen/progestogen therapy be managed?

It is important to remember that with combination therapies the incidence of endometrial cancer observed in large-scale, epidemiological studies has never been zero, and some women still develop endometrial malignancy.

As discussed in Question 6.35, the incidence of endometrial hyperplasia is related to the duration of progestogen addition and even with an adequate daily dose is 3–4% with 7 days of progestogen each month/cycle, and 2–3% with 10 days of progestogen addition. When prescribed for the currently recommended 12 days each month/cycle, endometrial hyperplasia can still arise if the daily progestogen dose is inadequate. The development of endometrial hyperplasia with a combined therapy indicates an inadequate progestational stimulus, irrespective of cause. While the majority of endometrial hyperplasias revert to normal endometrium when an adequate progestational stimulus is subsequently applied, some do not.

Although the data are sparse, the failure of reversion to normal endometrium is more likely with atypical hyperplasia.

Because of the lack of universal reversion, we believe it necessary to perform a further D&C after 4–6 months of an adequate course of progestogen. We prescribe the progestogen in 21-day courses. Failure of reversion is an indication for hysterectomy.

9.44 What is the value of endometrial ablation/resection in patients with heavy withdrawal bleeding in the absence of intrauterine pathology?

This is not known because the required studies have not been performed. In theory, it may be of value in the patient with chronic, heavy withdrawal bleeding in whom intrauterine pathology has been excluded. However, we think it wise, after ablation (or resection) to continue to prescribe a combined oestrogen/progestogen regimen. This is because endometrial ablation cannot guarantee to destroy 100% of endometrial tissue, and the progestogen should be continued to protect the small area of endometrium which may remain after ablation/resection surgery.

A long-term disadvantage of endometrial ablation is that it may cause intrauterine adhesions. Further D&C, for any indication, may then be impossible.

9.45 What effect may HRT have on endometriosis?

Endometriosis is an oestrogen-dependent condition and may be exacerbated by HRT or re-activated if dormant. Patients who have undergone total abdominal hysterectomy and bilateral salpingo-oophorectomy with complete excision of all endometriotic tissue are currently believed to be at low risk from a recurrence if they take HRT. However, if excision of the endometriosis was incomplete then HRT can reactivate dormant disease.

We have a series of patients (data unpublished), some of whom had undergone hysterectomy and bilateral salpingo-oophorectomy, in whom endometriosis has been re-activated with HRT in the following sites: the ovary, the adnexae and pelvic side-wall, the top of the vagina and the large bowel. The presenting complaints included pelvic pain, severe dysmenorrhoea and deep dyspareunia. In some, the passage of blood and/or mucus rectally was observed around the time of the withdrawal bleeding. There was a suggestion that one patient had developed hydronephrosis due to the re-activated endometriosis causing ureteric obstruction. The renal enlargement resolved when HRT was withdrawn. We have also observed a re-activation of endometriosis (requiring total abdominal hysterectomy and bilateral salpingo-oophorectomy) in a woman first starting HRT 12 years after menopause. Thus, there seems to be no upper time limit after menopause when HRT can be prescribed safely, and comments that it is safe to administer oestrogens 3–5 years after hysterectomy/menopause have, we believe, no scientific basis.

Patients with a history of endometriosis, especially those with residual disease, should be advised to stop HRT if they develop symptoms or signs suggestive of re-activation. We stress that the incidence of re-activation is most probably low but no data are currently available as to the precise risk. Thus, patients in whom endometriosis may be re-activated should be closely supervised with more frequent pelvic examinations, perhaps every 6–12 months. Pelvic ultrasonography may be helpful if symptoms and signs suggestive of re-activation occur.

9.46 If a patient has no withdrawal bleeding on sequential oestrogen/progestogen treatment how should she be managed?

Up to 15% of patients have no withdrawal bleeding on standard combined sequential oestrogen/progestogen HRT regimens. The incidence of amenorrhoea appears to increase with longer-term use of HRT; the withdrawal bleeding gradually diminishes from approximately 5 days to 2 days and then stops. There is no evidence that the absence of bleeding is harmful and current thinking is that no special investigations are necessary. Endometrial biopsy is not indicated. Amenorrhoea may result from complete suppression of endometrial growth by the added progestogen leading to an atrophic endometrium; an alternative explanation is that the oestrogen dose is insufficient to promote an endometrial response. However, most patients will still experience relief of symptoms. If the latter explanation is correct, it is unknown whether patients with amenorrhoea are receiving an adequate dose of oestrogen to prevent bone loss.

9.47 What other problems may arise on HRT?

Any medical condition can arise in HRT-users although it is rare to find that HRT is implicated in the aetiology. It would be impossible to provide a comprehensive review and we have limited ourselves to a discussion of the more common problems.

9.48 If hypertension develops should HRT be discontinued?

Not always. The risk of hypertension is related to many factors including age and body weight. Thus, it is almost inevitable that some users of HRT will develop idiopathic hypertension, especially if they are obese.

There is no good evidence that blood pressure is related to the stage of the ovulatory cycle, and that it increases around mid-cycle at the time of maximal oestradiol production in the non-pregnant female. Because the plasma oestradiol values achieved with oral and transdermal HRT (see Questions 6.5 and Figure 6.1) are lower than the pre-menopausal mid-cycle range (and thus lower than the levels achieved at ovulation), there seems no logical reason to incriminate moderate plasma oestradiol doses, achieved by these routes, in the genesis of hypertension. Additionally, recent research has shown that oestradiol acts as an arterial vasodilator, not as a vaso-constrictor (see Question 4.34).

Unlike non-oral oestrogens, it is well recognized that orally administered oestrogens increase renin substrate (see Chapter 6) and, in theory, they may thereby affect the renin–angiotensin axis. These differences between oral and non-orally administered oestrogens are discussed in Question 6.4 and illustrated in Figure 6.2. In summary, the forms of renin substrate induced by oral oestrogens have not been shown to be the forms of renin substrate associated with changes in blood pressure. Furthermore, the majority of women on oral oestrogens will increase their renin substrate levels but few, only 1–2%, develop clinically relevant hypertension. It has been suggested that increases in blood pressure during HRT are due more to an increase in weight than to the oestrogen; alternatively, it has been postulated that women developing hypertension represent a sub-group with an idiosyncratic response to oral oestrogens.

9.49 Can patients on antihypertensive medication receive HRT?

Yes. Well-controlled hypertension is not a contraindication to HRT. Patients should receive standard antihypertensive treatment and after the blood pressure is suitably controlled HRT can be commenced. In these circumstances, there is a theoretical advantage in the use of non-oral oestrogens, because they appear to cause less disturbances in the hepatic production of proteins and globulins which may be involved in the genesis of hypertension. We emphasize that at this time this is theoretical, and oral oestrogens have been shown to reduce the risk of arterial disease in hypertensive women (see Question 5.37 and Table 5.2).

It is generally accepted that repeated readings of blood pressure greater than 160/95 or 160/100 mmHg would be too high for starting HRT or continuing HRT without suitable antihypertensive medication.

9.50 Does HRT cause weight gain?

This was discussed in Question 7.3.

9.51 If a patient develops a breast lump should HRT be discontinued?

It would be normal practice to refer such a patient urgently for a surgical opinion. If the lump is subsequently shown to be malignant then most surgeons strongly advise that HRT should not be prescribed again. However, there are no data showing that the survival of patients with breast cancer is adversely affected by subsequent use of HRT; similarly, there are no data to show that it is influenced beneficially. Regrettably, the required studies have not been performed. (See also Question 8.1).

If the lump is shown to be benign (or if cyst aspiration shows no malignant cells), the patient will then have to decide whether or not to re-start HRT. The data from the National Cancer Institutes in the United States show that women developing surgically confirmed benign breast disease *after starting* HRT do not appear to be at an increase in risk of breast cancer. This applies even if the HRT is administered long-term for periods up to 10 years. Clearly, if the breast histology is of a condition (such as lobular or ductal hyperplasia) which carries a well recognized increase in lifetime risk of breast cancer, then the patient should be so notified and made aware of the desirability of increased surveillance. However, whether HRT will increase the risk further in this situation is not clear (see also Question 8.38).

9.52 How should a complaint of pain or cramp in the legs be managed?

There is no clear epidemiological evidence that natural oestrogens are associated with an increase in risk of superficial or deep venous thrombosis.

Careful assessment and examination are most important. As discussed in Question 7.2, leg cramps which occur in both calves and which tend to be worse during the night frequently occur during the first few weeks after starting HRT. The mechanism of action is unknown. In our studies using iodine [131]-labelled fibrinogen we were unable to demonstrate that such cramps were associated with thrombotic disease.

If symptoms are unilateral, a DVT must be excluded. Accurate diagnosis is most important and it is our belief that the patient should be referred for further investigation. All too frequently we see patients in whom DVT has been diagnosed on clinical grounds during HRT administration but in whom subsequent venograms (performed at our request) have been normal.

The decision to continue or discontinue HRT will depend upon whether DVT has or has not been demonstrated by appropriate investigations, such as venography or Doppler ultrasound flow studies.

9.53 Should HRT be discontinued prior to surgery?

It is a common belief that HRT should be discontinued both prior to elective surgery and at the time of emergency surgery. However, there is no evidence that this strategy reduces the risk of post-operative venous thrombotic disease. Furthermore, there is no evidence that HRT increases this risk.

As stated so many times during this book, contraceptive pill data should not be extrapolated to the use of natural oestrogens in postmenopausal women. The synthetic oestrogens (ethinyl oestradiol and mestranol) as used in the pill clearly cause changes in fibrinolytic and coagulation factors. The overwhelming majority of studies which have investigated the effects of oral natural oestrogens on these factors report no changes. One or two studies have reported adverse effects; one research group which so reported also studied the effects of the pill and concluded that the spectrum and severity of fibrinolytic and coagulation changes observed with oral HRT were less than those observed with the pill.

If the majority of the published studies are wrong and *if* (two big 'ifs') oral oestrogens in HRT cause clinically relevant fibrinolytic and coagulation changes, then how long prior to surgery should oral HRT be discontinued? We would argue that it may be some months. Certain changes in fibrinolytic and coagulation factors (Factor X; cephalin time and Factor VII) induced by the pill have been reported as taking up to 9 months to revert to normal after the pill is discontinued. Furthermore, recently published data on the pill indicate that discontinuation is followed by a rebound phenomenon. Thus, if oral HRT is clinically relevant with respect to post-operative venous thrombotic disease, we fail to see why discontinuing treatment only 1–2 weeks pre-operatively will remove the risk.

Non-orally administered oestradiol, via a patch, gives rise to plasma oestradiol levels in the mid-proliferative phase range. If such a plasma value significantly increased the risk of post-operative DVT and pulmonary embolism then all premenopausal women should undergo ovarian suppression prior to elective surgery. This, of course, does not happen because there is no evidence that plasma oestradiol values correlate with the risk of post-operative venous thrombosis. There is no excess risk in premenopausal women undergoing surgery around ovulation when plasma oestradiol values are highest. Thus, it seems illogical to incriminate transdermal oestradiol as a potential cause of an increase in risk of post-operative DVT and pulmonary embolism. Similar comments apply to other non-oral routes of oestradiol administration, such as subcutaneous implants.

In practice, the decision regarding continuation of HRT throughout the peri-operative period rests with the surgeon and anaesthetist caring for the patient. Despite the above comments, many doctors still adopt a cautious approach and recommend stopping HRT prior to elective major surgery and for minor surgery which involves immobilization (e.g. surgery for varicose veins). We do not stop HRT. Sudden discontinuation of HRT will involve the prompt return of symptoms but many doctors would argue that this is acceptable since the symptoms are not life-threatening. Others may be willing to allow a patient to remain on HRT containing natural oestrogens particularly when given via a non-oral route. However, the presence of other risk factors for thrombosis such as obesity and cigarette smoking may be more relevant than HRT.

9.54 How should jaundice which is caused by HRT be managed?

There is a rare condition in which an increase in the oestrogen environment is 'hepatotoxic'. The underlying mechanism is poorly understood but is believed to represent an idiosyncratic response. The result is cholestatic jaundice. This condition may be unmasked during pregnancy ('the fatty liver' of pregnancy) and can arise during the administration of the contraceptive pill. No data are available on the effects of HRT. In theory, non-oral routes of administration would be preferable because these minimize the amount of oestradiol presented to the liver as a 'bolus' (see Question 6.6).

Gilbert's syndrome in which bilirubin levels are elevated without jaundice (and the condition is usually only diagnosed on biochemical investigations) is not a contraindication to HRT.

The majority of oestrogen (approximately 90%) is degraded and metabolized within hepatic tissue. Presenting oestrogen to the liver at a time of disturbed function, such as jaundice, may be undesirable and we believe that HRT should be discontinued in patients with significant, active liver disease and jaundice. We see no reason why HRT should not be re-started when the liver function tests have returned to normal.

9.55 Does HRT cause gallstones?

It has been reported that oral natural oestrogens increase the risk of gallstones because they cause changes in the composition of bile. Thus, HRT must be used with great caution in such patients. It is not known whether transdermal oestradiol causes less changes in bile composition and therefore could be used with close supervision.

Patients who have undergone cholecystectomy may use HRT again.

9.56 Does HRT aggravate migraine?

The relationships between oestrogens, progesterone and progestogens and migraine are poorly understood.

It is possible that *menstrual* migraine (which starts 24–48 hours prior to the onset of menstruation) may result from the fall in plasma oestradiol that occurs at this time, and there are reports that menstrual migraine is improved by an oestrogen supplement (see Question 5.18). Whether a similar aetiology applies to *premenstrual* migraine, which may start 4–5 days before menstruation, is not clear; this could equally well result from the influence of progesterone.

Because of these uncertainties, the response of women who have suffered with menstrual and premenstrual migraine during the reproductive era to HRT is unpredictable. There is no alternative to a trial of therapy if the woman wishes to take HRT. She should be warned that migraine may return during or towards the end of the phase of progestogen addition. If it does then trying different types of progestogens is often of limited value because, in our experience, all progestogens appear to produce similar adverse responses with respect to migraine.

Curiously, some women who have not suffered with migraine during the reproductive era develop migraine-like headaches during the climacteric and in the early postmenopausal years. This group of patients is usually helped by HRT. The mechanism of action is unknown but may be through oestrogens influencing arterial wall tone (see Question 4.34).

10. Duration of therapy

At present, there are no universally accepted recommendations regarding the most appropriate duration of HRT. For most indications, there is a consensus among the majority of specialists in the field. The areas where disagreement exists will be clearly defined.

10.1 Who should make the decision about duration of therapy?

The decision should be taken jointly by the patient and her doctor. In symptomatic women the duration of therapy is dictated more by the type of symptom than by its severity (see Question 10.4). In asymptomatic women taking HRT to reduce the later risk of osteoporotic fractures and, perhaps, arterial disease risk, only approximate guidelines on the duration of therapy can be issued at present. This is because information on how the duration of HRT reduces the risk of these diseases (see Questions 10.5 and 10.6) remains incomplete.

Both parties must be aware that the indications for continuing with HRT may change with time. For example, the woman who has taken HRT because of troublesome hot flushes and night sweats may be successfully weaned off treatment after 2 years and the vasomotor symptoms may not return. However, she may present at a later date requesting further HRT to relieve troublesome vaginal dryness. Alternatively, during a course of HRT perhaps prescribed for relief of vasomotor symptoms, a woman's elder sister or mother may have sustained an osteoporotic fracture. The patient, although no longer symptomatic, may then elect to continue with HRT to prevent postmenopausal bone loss. As discussed elsewhere, there are numerous areas where our current knowledge about the long-term effects of HRT are deficient, and as the results of further research become available they may change the balance of perceived benefits and risks. Thus, the doctor will need to be a continuing source of information.

10.2 What will determine the patient's views?

In general, the patient will wish to continue with treatment if the perceived benefits outweigh the disadvantages. This is the most important determinant.

As previously stated, the majority of women currently taking HRT do so to alleviate troublesome vasomotor symptoms, psychological problems or symptoms arising from atrophy of the lower genital tract. A minority take HRT to prevent osteoporosis and to reduce the risk of arterial disease. In both groups, the disadvantages of HRT are greater for women who have an intact uterus as compared to women who have undergone hysterectomy. The continuation or return of monthly 'periods' is regarded by many women as a disadvantage despite the fact that the bleeding should not be heavy or painful and tends to become lighter as the duration of HRT is extended. The other side-effects of progestogen therapy, such as breast tenderness, depression, anxiety and irritability (see Question 7.8) may dissuade some women from continuing with HRT, although it is often possible to reduce the frequency and severity of these side-effects by altering the type or dose of progestogen (see Questions 7.9 and 7.10).

The importance of various other factors, which we suspect is considerable, has not been adequately determined. While some women are keen to undergo regular examination, other women may discontinue therapy because they dislike making regular visits to a doctor or nurse. Regrettably, because 'bad news' seems to attract more publicity than good news, adverse reports about the effect of any therapy seem to achieve a higher media profile than favourable reports. Thus, some women may discontinue therapy in response to a 'scare' media report or adverse comments from relatives or friends.

Some women may decide to stop therapy because of symptoms which they wrongly attribute to HRT, e.g. excessive weight gain, constipation etc.

10.3 What will determine the doctor's views?

We suspect that these will be medical, administrative and financial.

The benefits, side-effects and risks of HRT have been comprehensively discussed elsewhere in this book. In the overwhelming majority of patients it will be possible to find a treatment regimen which maximises benefits yet causes minimal side-effects. The major anxiety with HRT is the effect of long-term therapy on breast cancer risk. These data are contradictory and at variance (see Question 8.35). Those doctors who believe that a causal relationship has yet to be established beyond all reasonable doubt often recommend that therapy can be given for periods of up to 20 years or even lifelong; those who believe that a causal relationship has been established are much more cautious and often recommend that HRT should not be prescribed for durations of more than 5 years unless a strong indication is present.

The one group of patients in which all authorities agree that long-term treatment with HRT is desirable is women with premature menopause, or prolonged periods of hypo-oestrogenism during the reproductive era (see Questions 5.4–5.13).

Expensive equipment is not required to monitor the effects of HRT. Prescribing HRT will increase the workload of the primary care physician, but some of this can be delegated to a suitably trained, practice nurse (see Questions 11.4 and 11.5). Whether this increase in the workload of the primary care physician will be offset by a greater reduction in use of primary care and other national health service resources (e.g. care because of osteoporotic fracture, myocardial infarction or cerebrovascular accident) is not known. Furthermore, it is not clear whether HRT will be cost-effective. The currently available analyses on cost-benefit suggest that oestrogen-only treatments are cost-effective, but that combination oestrogen/progestogen therapies are not. This difference has arisen because the latter are more expensive, and also because it has been assumed in these analyses that combined treatments will afford only one half of the protection of oestrogen-only therapy in reducing arterial disease risk. It is emphasized that this is an assumption which may be erroneous (see Questions 4.36 and 8.45).

We believe that it is too early to draw any financial conclusions about the effect of the recommendations in the White Paper. However, we hope that the availability of HRT and other therapies will not be constrained by the costs of drugs, equipment or staff.

10.4 What is the recommended duration of therapy for a patient with symptoms?

As discussed in Question 3.6, while the typical symptoms of vasomotor instability are self-limiting to a degree, it is important to remember that 70% of women who suffer vasomotor disturbances do so for up to 2 years, and up to 25% will experience these symptoms for 5 years. A few, perhaps 5%, may have these symptoms very long-term, up to 20 years. The percentage of women experiencing psychological problems for long periods is not known but is likely to be similar. Therefore, for most women the minimum duration of therapy for relief of these symptoms should be 2–3 years. Therapy can then be withdrawn (see Question 10.9). Some women will experience a recurrence of these symptoms and they may request a further course of HRT. In these circumstances a longer duration of therapy, perhaps 5 years in total, will be required. A small number of women may need very long-term treatment.

The percentage of women experiencing symptoms due to atrophy of the lower genital tract increases with time since menopause (see Questions 3.31–3.35). Women with symptoms due to lower urogenital tract atrophy may require very long-term treatment, especially if their dyspareunia and urethral problems are only effectively alleviated by oestrogens. Our longest users of HRT are women in this group.

Until recently, the average duration of a course of HRT has been only 3 months in the UK. Although this has now risen to 6 months, even this falls short of the above recommendations. We believe that it is illogical to prescribe HRT for a few months and then to stop it just when patients are beginning to feel better. We do not think that this practice can be justified, especially as it may cause considerable patient distress. Initially, women do not understand why further treatment is withheld. If they are told that the reasons for stopping treatment are concerns about safety, particularly cancer, then women often become alarmed and feel that they may have caused long-term damage to themselves. Patients who find HRT to be beneficial can be reassured that it has a good safety profile when administered for periods of up to 5 years (see Question 8.45 and Table 8.8). Longer-term therapy may be justified but the risk/benefit ratio will need to be reviewed on a regular basis (see Question 10.1).

10.5 What is the recommended duration of therapy for a patient who wishes to prevent osteoporotic fractures?

It is generally accepted that 5 years of HRT prescribed soon after menopause will reduce the risk of fracture of the vertebral body and hip by approximately 50% (see Question 4.22). Data on the fracture risk from longer-term studies are sparse. However, it would not be surprising if 10 years of HRT prescribed soon after menopause reduced vertebral fracture risk by as much as 75%. Data on the value of HRT in reducing the risk of fracture in older women are even more sparse (see Question 4.21).

10.6 What is the recommended duration of therapy for patients wishing to reduce their risk of arterial disease?

Again, the epidemiological data are sparse. Beneficial effects have been observed within 2–3 years of starting HRT. Unlike the reduction in risk of osteoporotic fracture, the current belief is that HRT does not exert a duration-dependent protection against arterial disease risk, and the observed reductions in risk of between 30% and 70% apply equally to women taking HRT in their 50s and also in their 70s. Sparse data suggest that some of the protective effect is lost within 2 years of discontinuing treatment (see Question 4.40).

10.7 Does a patient's age at menopause alter the recommended duration of therapy?

The particular problems of women with premature menopause and prolonged periods of amenorrhoea associated with hypo-oestrogenism during the reproductive era were discussed in Questions 5.4–5.13. To avoid the early development of osteoporotic fractures and arterial disease, it has been recommended that such women receive HRT until age 50 years. Whether treatment should then be continued further in this group, perhaps until age 60 or 65 years, is not known and we believe that a careful assessment of the benefit/risk ratio will be required on an individual basis.

The benefits of oestrogens when started in women many years after menopause on osteoporotic fracture and arterial disease risk have been referred to above, and were comprehensively discussed in Questions 4.21 and 4.37.

10.8 Is it true that once a patient has been commenced on HRT she will need to take it for the rest of her life?

No. Patients taking HRT for symptomatic relief can often be successfully weaned off therapy if the symptom was self-limiting (vasomotor disturbances; psychological symptoms). Patients with symptoms which are not self-limiting (lower genital tract problems) invariably experience a recurrence of their symptoms after oestrogens are withdrawn.

10.9 How should HRT be discontinued?

Abrupt cessation of HRT often results in an exacerbation of hot flushes, night sweats and psychological symptoms. Therefore, therapy should be tailed off gradually over a period of 2–3 months. In patients taking oral therapy the dosage should first be reduced to the lowest strength tablet (e.g.

patients taking conjugated equine oestrogens 1.25 mg/day should be changed to 0.625 mg/day). After 3−4 weeks on the lowest dose tablet an alternate-day regimen is introduced for another 3−4 weeks, and finally patients are advised to extend the duration between tablets (to 4 or 5 days) for another 2 weeks and then to stop therapy completely.

Similar comments apply to patients using transdermal oestradiol therapy. The oestradiol dose can be gradually reduced from 100 μg/day through 50 μg/day to 25 μg/day. Following this, patients are advised to introduce a treatment-free break between patches starting with 1−2 days and gradually increasing this until the lowest strength patch is only worn for 3 days every 7−10 days. Treatment can then be stopped.

It is always worthwhile warning patients that hot flushes, night sweats and psychological problems may recur during the weaning-off process. Often, these are not frequent nor severe; if they are, then the patient will either have to tolerate them or return to therapy. Because the frequency and severity of vasomotor disturbances appears to be influenced by the ambient temperature, we do not routinely wean patients off therapy who initially presented with these symptoms during the summer months, and we try to discontinue therapy during the winter. Again, anecdotally, we do not wean patients off therapy who initially presented with psychological problems at times of stress (for many women the 6 weeks before Christmas appears stressful and we avoid this).

The need for progestogen addition in women with an intact uterus is debatable during withdrawal of oral and transdermal oestrogens. Some authorities recommend that an adequate dose of progestogen be continued during this phase, but others do not. If a progestogen is administered then the patient should be warned that the withdrawal bleeding is likely to become much lighter and scantier, or that it may cease completely as the oestrogen dose is reduced. Many women experience a light withdrawal bleed of approximately 2−3 days' duration when therapy is finally stopped.

10.10 Is it more difficult to tail off implant therapy?

It can be. We have already referred to the high (and sometimes supra-physiological) plasma oestradiol levels that can be achieved with implant therapy (see Question 6.16). Because endometrial stimulation may be achieved with plasma oestradiol values above 200 pmol/l, and because it may take many months (if not years) for the plasma oestradiol values to return to below this level after last implantation, we believe that progestogen addition should be continued for an appropriate duration each month (preferably 12 days) following last implantation until amenorrhoea occurs in 3 consecutive months following progestogen administration.

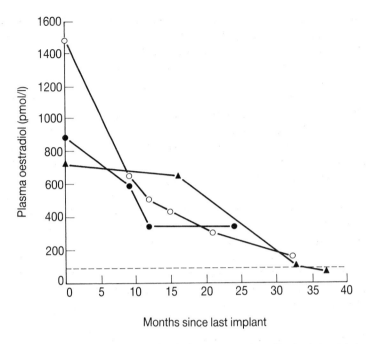

Fig. 10.1   Plasma oestradiol concentrations in three women at time of last implant and during follow-up period. ▲ =case 2, O = case 5, ● =case 7, --- = Postmenopausal range (<100 pmol/l) (From Gangar K F, Fraser D, Whitehead M I, Cust M P. 1990 British Medical Journal 300: 436–438. Reproduced with permission.)

Figure 10.1 shows the gradual decline in plasma oestradiol levels that was observed following last implantation in three patients; it was between 30 and 40 months before withdrawal bleeding ceased. Table 10.1 gives details of a series of patients who continued to experience withdrawal bleeding for periods of between 12 and 43 months after last implantation. Table 10.1 also gives details of the total duration of implant therapy and the average annual dose. In no patient was this excessive (less than 108 mg oestradiol per annum). Because chronic, unopposed oestrogen stimulation can result in endometrial neoplasia, we think it important that patients with an intact uterus who have been treated with oestradiol implants be advised to continue with the progestogen on a monthly basis until all endometrial stimulation has ceased. In our practice, we recommend that the progestogen be continued until administration has failed to produce a withdrawal bleed in 3 consecutive months.

Table 10.1 Details of oestradiol implant therapy, reasons for discontinuing treatment, and duration of withdrawal bleeding in 10 postmenopausal women following last implantation.

Case number	Total oestradiol dose (mg)	Time between first and last implants	Average oestradiol dose (mg/year)	Reason for discontinuing implant treatment	Duration of withdrawal bleeding (months) until final event	Age at end of observation period (years)
1	350	3 years 2 months	96	Progestogen intolerance	43*	57
2	150	1 year 3 months	86	No symptoms	40*	60
3	150	1 year 1 month	95	No symptoms	30*	52
4	225	3 years	64	Breast carcinoma	27*	59
5	225	2 years 3 months	82	Breakthrough bleeding with atypical hyperplasia	26†	60
6	375	3 years	107	No symptoms	36‡	54
7	325	4 years 6 months	65	No symptoms	30‡	42
8	100	6 months	100	No symptoms	22‡	49
9	325	3 years 6 months	81	No symptoms but atypical hyperplasia	21§	68
10	150	2 years 2 months	56	Worry about breast cancer	12§	59

* Ceased bleeding spontaneously.
† Withdrawal bleeding continued until hysterectomy.
‡ Withdrawal bleeding continued until oestrogen treatment restarted.
§ Continued regular withdrawal bleeding.
(From Gangar K F, Fraser D, Whitehead M I, Cust M P 1990 British Medical Journal 300: 436–438. Reproduced with permission.)

10.11 Are attempts to withdraw patients from HRT always successful?

No. Despite careful attempts to withdraw HRT some patients will experience a recurrence of troublesome symptoms (usually vasomotor disturbances and psychological problems) and will want to resume HRT. Patients with symptoms due to lower genital tract atrophy can expect these to return if HRT is withdrawn, although the interval may be some months. Additionally, some patients taking HRT because of flushes, sweats and/or psychological problems do not experience these symptoms when treatment is stopped but return at a later date complaining of lower genital tract symptoms.

10.12 Can patients take HRT indefinitely?

Yes. Women who are satisfied with treatment and feel well on it often want to continue. Inevitably, women who have undergone hysterectomy constitute a large part of this group. Women who find their monthly periods troublesome and the progestogenic side-effects unacceptable are more likely to discontinue HRT.

The major concern about the long-term use of HRT revolves around the risk of breast cancer (see Question 8.34). We believe that patients should be made aware that some research studies have shown an increase in risk with very long-term use of HRT but that this is controversial.

10.13 Are there any methods of predicting when HRT can be stopped?

As far as relief of vasomotor disturbances and psychological problems is concerned, the majority of patients will find that 2–3 years of HRT will be adequate. However, 25% of women with these symptoms experience them for 5 years and they may need treatment for this long. As yet, there are no methods of predicting which patients will require longer-term therapy. Unfortunately, this may only be resolved by assessment of the response to withdrawal of HRT.

10.14 Are there any conditions when HRT should be discontinued, either permanently or temporarily?

These are discussed in Questions 9.47–9.56.

11. Running a clinic in general practice

During the last decade, primary care physicians have spent an increasing amount of time trying to prevent illness relative to that spent treating established disease. For example, most now appreciate the value of screening for and treating hypertension, and recognize the benefits of advising patients on risk factors such as smoking and excessive alcohol consumption. Under the terms of the new contract of 1990, the balance between anticipatory and reactive care is likely to shift even further in favour of screening.

Running a menopause clinic involves both anticipatory and reactive care. The provision and monitoring of HRT within the framework of a Well Woman/Health Promotion Clinic can result in a comprehensive counselling and screening service for climacteric women; such a service, if well organized, is much appreciated by patients and rewarding for the staff involved. Most patients who take HRT can be successfully managed within primary care; only rarely is hospital referral necessary, unless there are special contraindications to or significant problems with HRT.

11.1 What should be the aims of a Menopause Clinic?

The principal aims are as follows:

1. Provision of information and advice
2. Relief of distressing symptoms
3. Prevention of osteoporosis
4. Reduction of ischaemic heart disease and strokes.

However, a Menopause Clinic provides ideal opportunities for:

1. Screening, e.g. breast cancer, cervical cancer, hypertension, diabetes, hyperlipidaemia

2. Health education, e.g. diet, exercise, anti-smoking, alcohol control, stress management
3. Training, e.g. medical students, GP vocational trainees, nurses, health visitors, etc.
4. Research.

11.2 What are the steps involved in setting up such a clinic?

The 10 basic steps are summarized in Table 11.1

Table 11.1 Ten basic steps in setting up a Menopause Clinic

1. staff employment and training
2. construction of age/sex register
3. review of premises for space and equipment
4. arrangement of clinic sessions within surgery timetable
5. development of clinic protocol and submission to FHSA for approval as health promotion clinic (to attract fees)
6. establish record system and ensure adequate follow-up of results with patient call/recall system
7. obtaining educational literature
8. recruiting patients
    - practice leaflet
    - opportunistic
    - systematic (letter of invitation)
9. establish telephone 'helpline' service
10. establish audit system (including FHSA returns, form FP/HPC)

11.3 What staff will be required?

An enthusiastic doctor and nurse (or health visitor) are the basic minimum requirements. A sympathetic team is essential. It has been shown that women benefit greatly from having their problems treated seriously and sympathetically. This may be the principal reason why women self-refer to hospital menopause clinics.

A clinic receptionist will be useful to ease the administrative load. In the long-term, a counsellor would be a valuable addition to the team for those patients with mid-life problems (including psycho-sexual difficulties) not related to oestrogen deficiency.

11.4 What qualifications are necessary for practice nurses working in a Well Woman/Health Promotion/Menopause Clinic?

Most practice nurses are registered general nurses (RGN) and have attended a basic practice nursing course.

No additional formal qualifications are required. A nurse with experience in family planning clinics, cervical cytology clinics or gynaecology outpatient clinics would be a bonus. Experience in clinics allied to the Oxford Prevention of Heart Attack and Stroke Project would also be useful. Many health visitors have experience of health promotion work, counselling and stress management.

In reality, a caring, sympathetic nature and enthusiasm for the job are all that are required. Any mismatch between practice requirements and the nurse's knowledge and skills can be rectified by training.

11.5 What training courses are available?

Courses are available for family planning training, including cervical cytology and breast screening. Courses are also available from the Oxford Prevention of Heart Attack and Stroke Project together with national practice nurse conferences.

Further information about nurse training courses on the menopause are available from the Amarant Trust (see page 224).

11.6 How can the potential workload be assessed?

The target population will be women aged 40 (or 45) to 60 years of age. The numbers can be assessed from the Practice Age Sex Register. A practice of 10 000 patients will contain approximately 1400 women aged between 40 and 60 years.

The amount of time involved per consultation will have to be tailored according to the available resources. Ideally 20–30 minutes would be an appropriate time for an initial consultation. We appreciate that this may be impossible but we again emphasize that the advisability of prescribing HRT, or otherwise, is influenced by many factors. These include not only details of the patient's medical history, but also factors in the family history (breast cancer, osteoporosis, arterial disease). The use of the practice nurse as an aide in history-taking and examination was discussed in Questions 9.7–9.9.

Subsequent visits require much shorter periods of time.

11.7 What are the requirements on premises?

It is highly unlikely that any additional premises will be required. The doctor and nurse will both require a room for consultations. An examination/treatment room will be required as will a waiting area for the patients.

11.8 What equipment is necessary?

No special equipment is required in addition to that which should already be available in a practice offering family planning/cervical cytology services.

11.9 When should clinics be held?

Local needs may vary as will the availability of staff, time and space.

Most women in full-time employment will prefer to attend clinics held in the evenings. Some women, however, will be able to attend morning or afternoon sessions. Thus, one Well Woman Clinic session could be held during the morning or afternoon, and a second could be held during the evening, each week. Menopause Clinic sessions could be held every other week, perhaps alternating with family planning sessions.

11.10 How should a clinic protocol be established?

Good teamwork is essential. The roles of the doctor and nurse should complement each other.

The steps involved in establishing a clinical protocol are as follows:

1. The responsibilities of the GP and practice nurse should be clearly defined.

2. A structured plan of care should be devised so that every patient passing through the clinic receives the same level of advice, assessment, investigation, treatment and follow-up.

3. Initial history-taking and screening can be performed by the nurse. To assist with this, the patient can complete a questionnaire providing background information on her past history and present symptoms, and on the family history.

4. The doctor should perform an initial assessment of the patient as described in Questions 5.1, 5.2, 9.7, 9.10 and 9.12.

5. No additional examinations are usually required in the pre-HRT screen beyond those that should routinely be performed on a woman of that age.

6. No additional investigations are required in normal, healthy women with no specific risk factors.

7. Every patient should have a record card to indicate attendance at the clinic, to document findings, to record details of treatment and to ensure proper follow-up.

8. The first follow-up visit is usually after 3 months with further clinic visits at 12–18 monthly intervals thereafter (see Questions 9.27–9.28). A computerized call/recall system is useful but not essential.

9. Patients should be encouraged to return to the clinic for regular monitoring.

10. Patients should be instructed whom to contact if they require further advice (for example, if they experience side-effects). The availability of an experienced practice nurse, even for 2 hours each week for telephone counselling, can be invaluable.

11.11 How can patients be recruited to Well Women/ Health Promotion/Menopause Clinics?

In one or more of several ways:

1. The practice leaflet. Menopause counselling services and the provision of HRT can be listed under the heading of the Well Woman/Health Promotion Clinic. The timing of clinic sessions and the staff available should be stated under the same heading.

Practice leaflets are compulsory under the new contract of 1990. Because all registered patients will be receiving the literature, women will be made aware of your service.

2. Opportunistic screening. When the patient attends on another matter the opportunity can be taken to offer the services of the Well Woman/Health Promotion/Menopause Clinic. It should be remembered that 70% of the practice population will consult the primary care physician in one year and 90% in five years.

3. True screening. Patients can be actively pursued by means of personal invitations by letter to attend the Well Woman/Health Promotion/Menopause Clinic.

4. Posters can be displayed in the patient waiting area and nurse treatment room.

5. One can always rely on word of mouth!

11.12 Why do patients attend a Menopause Clinic?

These were discussed in Question 9.2. In summary, Menopause Clinic attenders usually fall into one or more of the following four categories:

1. Women seeking further information regarding the consequences of menopause, the role of HRT and its possible relevance to them.

2. Symptomatic patients with problems unequivocably due to oestrogen deficiency.

3. Symptomatic patients who believe (sometimes mistakenly) that their problems are due to oestrogen deficiency.

4. Asymptomatic patients. Women who seek advice regarding their risk of osteoporosis and/or heart disease and whether or not they should consider HRT.

As indicated previously (see Question 9.3) more women initially obtain information about HRT from the mass media or from a friend than from a health care professional.

11.13 What patient education material is available and where may it be obtained?

Books, booklets, audio and video cassettes etc., are available from sources listed in Appendix 2, page 224. In addition, many pharmaceutical companies provide patient education literature.

11.14 What is the role of the practice nurse in the Menopause Clinic?

There can be a spectrum of involvement for the practice nurse. This can range from clinics which are primarily doctor-based with minimal nursing assistance through to equal participation of the doctor and the nurse, although they will have different responsibilities. Those of the practice nurse can be summarized thus:

1. Assist with history-taking (see Questions 9.7 and 9.8).

2. Assist with the general examination (weight, blood pressure – see Question 9.10).
3. Explain the treatment to patients (see Question 9.25).
4. In patients with an intact uterus, explain when withdrawal bleeding may occur (see Question 9.25).
5. Provide telephone help-line advice (see Question 9.25).
6. Organize a call/recall system.
7. Monitor laboratory reports and follow-up, where required.
8. Organize patient education literature.
9. Liaise with self-help groups, etc.

In addition, the practice nurse can provide general health education advice (diet, reduction in cigarette and alcohol consumption, exercise, etc.).

11.15 What additional resources may be required?

Access to telephone advice is a very useful additional resource in the Menopause Clinic. Patients frequently require information or advice between clinic sessions. The service can be provided by an appropriately trained nurse and opportunities for patients to obtain telephone advice should be available, at least during office hours (see also Question 9.25).

11.16 How can the costs of running a Menopause Clinic be offset?

Under the terms of the new 1990 contract, a sessional fee will be paid to primary care physicians organizing Well Woman/Health Promotion Clinics (Form FP/MPC). A Menopause Clinic can be included as part of Well Woman screening and thereby should satisfy the requirements for a Health Promotion Clinic. Additionally, a Menopause Clinic provides an opportunity for cervical cancer screening. Many women who may not otherwise take up the invitation to have a cervical smear may be encouraged to attend a Menopause Clinic, thereby helping to achieve the cervical screening target for the practice.

Additional income can be generated from item-of-service fees e.g. tetanus vaccination and contraceptive advice.

12. Contraception

The contraceptive needs of a woman at any age who is either pre- or perimenopausal are, strictly speaking, beyond the terms of reference of this volume which deals specifically with HRT. Therefore, this chapter is in two parts: the first is a brief review of fertility and contraceptive requirements in women in these groups and we emphasize that more comprehensive information is available elsewhere (see *Contraception: Your Questions Answered*, Guillebaud in Guide to further reading); the second part deals with HRT and its relationship with contraception in the pre- and perimenopausal woman.

12.1 How fertile are 'older women'?

Whilst it is generally accepted that fertility declines with advancing age, precise statistics are hard to find.

There is a decline in fertility in most women during the late 30s through into the early 40s; it is often stated that the fertility of a woman around 40 years of age is half that of a 25-year-old. Part of this decline is due to the ageing ovary becoming progressively more refractory to gonadotrophin stimulation, and fertility appears to decline further as the perimenopause is approached. This has been recognized for many years by in-vitro fertilization (IVF) programmes, and many are reluctant to accept women over 40 years of age for IVF treatment. The precise mechanisms responsible for ovarian refractoriness are not known.

Another factor often cited as contributing to the decline in female fertility with advancing age is decreased coital frequency. However, this may not apply in newly formed relationships which, because of the increasing divorce rate, are no longer that uncommon in this age group.

Age-related data on the failure rate of various methods of contraception are available. However, age-banding has been very broad and, as far as the older woman is concerned, has been somewhat imprecise. For example, some studies have considered all women aged over 35 years as one group. We suspect that greater division into sub-groups by 5-year age-bands (35−39, 40−44, and 45−49 years) would have resulted in too few observations in the various age categories for meaningful analysis. However, the dearth of valid, comparative data on failure rates with certain methods of contraception between women in their late-30s as compared with those in their late-40s means that imprecise advice may be given to the older woman. Although of limited value to the perimenopausal woman, data on failure rates with certain forms of contraceptives are as shown in Table 12.1; the age-bands are indicated.

Because of the age-related decline in female fertility, a contraceptive method which is unacceptable to a younger woman of full fecundity may be acceptable to an older woman of diminished fertility. Thus, the progestogen-only 'mini' pill may be unacceptable to the younger age group, but perfectly acceptable to perimenopausal women.

The majority of women aged between 40 and 55 years with regular menstrual cycles appear to ovulate in every cycle. Changes in the menstrual pattern may indicate that the cycles are more likely to be anovulatory. Whilst ovulation itself does not correlate precisely with fertility, many women in their late-40s who are still menstruating appear to regard themselves, erroneously, as infertile and, therefore, there is a need for health education and contraceptive advice in this older age group.

12.2 Why is contraception so important?

The incidence of many of the well-recognized causes of maternal morbidity and mortality (e.g. pregnancy-induced hypertension, abruption) is increased in older women. Certain chromosomal abnormalities of the fetus (e.g. trisomy 21) are also more common.

Unwanted pregnancy often results in psychological trauma and this, in our limited experience, can be more marked in the older woman especially if she has a growing family. The happy experiences of pregnancy, childbirth and breastfeeding may be rekindled; however, there is often a sense of shame ('how can I now tell my teen-age daughter to be careful?'), and often there is also a sense of frustration ('how could I have been so stupid?'). The latter may be particularly marked if the prospects for peace and quiet (after the children had left home in the near future) were attractive.

12.3 For how long must contraception be continued after the menopause?

The menopause signals the end of the reproductive era, but the diagnosis can only be made in retrospect. Ovulation can occur up to the menopause. Women with climacteric symptoms including oligomenorrhoea and

Table 12.1 User-failure rates for various methods of contraceptives per 100 woman-years

Method	Age	
	25–34 years	35 years and over
Combined oral contraceptive pill	0.38	0.23
Progestogen-only pill	2.5	0.5
Diaphragm	5.5	2.8
Male sterilization	0.08	0.0
Female sterilization	0.45	0.08
Condom	4.4	3.1 (age 35–39) 1.5 (age 40–44)
Copper-7 IUCD	3.1	0.6
Short Multiload IUCD	2.4 (under 30 years)	0.5 (age 30 and over)

(Sources: Vessey M, Lawless M, Yeates D 1982 Lancet i: 841–842; Vessey M P, Villard-Mackintosh L, McPherson K, Yeates D 1988 British Journal of Family Planning 14: 40–43; UK Family Planning Research Network 1989 British Journal of Family Planning 15: 80–82. Reproduced with permission.)

amenorrhoea of up to 6-months' duration may have one further fertile ovulation leading to pregnancy.

Therefore it is recommended that contraception should be continued for 1 year after the last menstrual period if the woman is aged over 50 years, and for a further 2 years if she is aged under 50 years.

12.4 What is the best contraceptive method?

There is no single 'best' method for all women aged over 40 years. Couples must be assessed according to their own circumstances, and their wishes must be taken into account.

Although many couples opt for a 'permanent' method, such as sterilization, others prefer to avoid surgery and request information about the hormonal and non-hormonal alternatives.

12.5 At what age should the combined oral contraceptive be stopped?

The available data suggest that low-dose, combined oral contraceptives may be prescribed to fit, healthy, non-smokers who request them (and who have no cardiovascular risk factors) up to the age of 40 years. However, some doctors feel that the newer pills, such as those containing lower doses of ethinyl oestradiol (20 μg) and/or the most recently introduced, less androgenic progestogens (gestodene, desogestrel) can be prescribed to women up to the age of 45 years or even up to 50 years, the time of the menopause. We emphasize that no large-scale studies of combined oral contraceptive formulations have been performed in women aged up to 45 or 50 years. Despite this, in October 1989 the Fertility and Maternal Health Drugs Advisory Committee of the USA Food and Drug Administration (FDA) recommended to the FDA that there should be no upper limit for combined oral contraceptive use by healthy, non-smoking women.

Current thinking is that the combined pill should be discontinued at the age of 35 years in women who have risk factors for cardiovascular disease and especially those women who smoke.

12.6 If the combined oral contraceptive is prescribed to women in their forties, will it mask symptoms and signs of ovarian failure?

Yes. Because all combined pills contain an oestrogen they will suppress the development of symptoms and signs of ovarian failure. The oestrogen in all combined pills is either ethinyl oestradiol or mestranol (which is metabolized to ethinyl oestradiol) and both are administered at relatively high dosage when compared with the doses of 'natural' oestrogens which are used in modern HRT formulations. It is to be remembered that oral contraceptives are prescribed to achieve a pharmacological effect (suppression of ovulation); HRT is prescribed to achieve a physiological effect (replacement of oestrogens lost because of ovarian failure). Women taking the combined oral contraceptive will continue to experience regular 'periods' for as long as the pill is administered and, thus, the date of the 'natural' menopause will be masked.

12.7 Are HRT preparations contraceptive?

Modern combined HRT oestrogen/progestogen preparations do not suppress ovulation and are not contraceptive since the doses of the natural oestrogens used are too low. High doses of oral natural oestrogens may suppress ovulation e.g. conjugated equine oestrogens 7.5 mg/day, but such high doses have not been extensively investigated for contraceptive efficacy.

High doses of oestradiol from implants (perhaps 100 mg inserted every 6 months) or from patches (200 μg/day administered as two 100 μg patches) appear to suppress ovulation. However, few studies of these regimens as contraceptive agents have been performed. We think it premature to recommend these regimens for general contraceptive use at this time.

12.8 If a woman opts to continue with the combined oral contraceptive until around the time that 'natural' menopause would occur, at what time should she be switched from the 'combined pill' to an HRT preparation?

There is no satisfactory answer to this question which we have included because it is asked of us so frequently. However, the question assumes that following discontinuation of the oral contraceptive pill there will be an indication for HRT. A need for HRT may arise if, after stopping the combined pill, the woman develops typical menopausal symptoms. However, if these do not occur and she has no wish for preventative therapy should HRT be prescribed?

In our experience, many women continue the 'pill' into their late-40s not for contraceptive reasons but because of other benefits. For example, the 'pill' may have reduced or abolished premenstrual tension, improved dysmenorrhoea or controlled menorrhagia and many women have similar expectations of HRT. However, HRT does not suppress ovulation and therefore may not improve premenstrual tension or dysmenorrhoea nor, because the progestogen is added for only 12–13 days per month/cycle, may it control menorrhagia. Women should be disabused of unrealistic expectations of HRT.

Because of difficulties which may be experienced in synchronizing endogenous and exogenous steroid patterns, switching from the combined pill to HRT in perimenopausal women may cause cyclical symptoms of oestrogen excess and increase the risk of breakthrough bleeding (see Question 5.16). We would regard previous use of the combined pill as irrelevant and HRT should be instituted as described in Question 5.18.

In women in whom the combined pill has been used until the late-40s solely for contraceptive purposes the following options are available:

1. Discontinue the combined oral contraceptive pill at an arbitrary age (probably around the age of 50 years). If amenorrhoea ensues then an FSH assay can be performed 6–8 weeks later. A non-hormonal method of contraception must be used whilst these investigations are underway. Preferably, two FSH assays should be performed 4–8 weeks apart and if both show a level above 30 IU/l then ovarian failure, i.e. the postmenopausal phase, is strongly suggested. HRT can then be started if such therapy is requested for preventative reasons.

2. Discontinue the combined oral contraceptive and change to a non-hormonal method of contraception. Normal menstruation may return and the menopause occur naturally in due course. HRT may then be started if indicated.

3. Discontinue the combined pill and change to the progestogen-only 'mini' pill.

12.9 What advice should be given to women who commence HRT before their last 'natural' period?

The use of a modern HRT preparation in these circumstances will mask the date of the menopause. It is important to counsel the woman regarding her choice of contraceptive method before starting HRT in the pre- and perimenopausal phases.

Difficulties arise over the decision of when to discontinue contraceptive precautions when HRT is commenced in a woman before the menopause. Two strategies are available:

1. Discontinue the HRT preparation and assay the FSH level after 6–8 weeks. A value over 30 IU/l indicates the postmenopausal range, but a single raised FSH value may not guarantee complete absence of ovarian follicular activity or loss of fertility. Two raised FSH levels taken 4–8 weeks apart, together with amenorrhoea, would suggest significant loss of ovarian function. A non-hormonal contraceptive should be used for a further year (if the patient is over 50 years), or for a further 2 years (if the patient is under 50 years of age). This method of assessment is unpopular with patients as it necessitates the discontinuation of their HRT preparation and the return of their symptoms.

2. Continue HRT and the non-hormonal contraceptive method of choice until an arbitrary age has been attained. Here an assumption has to be made about the age at which fertility is lost, e.g. 55 years, but it is stressed that this is an assumption.

The stage at which all contraceptive precautions can safely be abandoned is indeterminate and, therefore, decisions can only be made on the balance of probabilities. Each woman will need individual assessment and guidance from her doctor. Those women who start HRT when premenopausal or early in the perimenopause and who elect to discontinue non-hormonal methods of contraception soon afterwards have to be prepared to take some responsibility for this decision since a guarantee that ovulation will not occur again cannot be given.

12.10 How useful is the progestogen-only pill?

Many women find this an acceptable method of contraception over the age of 35 years. The accidental pregnancy rate at the age of 35 years is approximately 0.8 per 100 woman-years, and 0.3 per 100 woman-years at 40 years and over.

Disadvantages include the strict pill-taking regimen required and poor cycle control, ranging from continuous spotting to amenorrhoea. Functional ovarian cysts are more common in progestogen-only pill users. There is no upper age limit to using the progestogen-only pill.

12.11 Does the use of the progestogen-only pill mask the date of the menopause?

It is unlikely that the dose of progestogen in the 'mini-pill' is sufficient to relieve vasomotor symptoms. Therefore, the onset of vasomotor symptoms in a woman taking the progestogen- only pill usually indicates that she is entering the climacteric. Unfortunately, the appearance of amenorrhoea cannot be taken as indicator of the climacteric. However, a raised FSH level on two separate occasions in these circumstances usually indicates ovarian failure and the woman should be advised to continue with contraceptive precautions for a further year if aged over 50 years, and for a further 2 years if aged under 50 years.

12.12 Can the progestogen-only pill be prescribed concurrently with a 'standard' cyclical combined oestrogen/progestogen HRT preparation?

Yes it can, and some doctors are doing so, *but* there are no data to support its use as a contraceptive in these circumstances. In fact, the presence of supplemental oestrogen may interfere with the action of the progestogen-only pill on the cervical mucus, a property which may be essential for its contraceptive efficacy.

12.13 Are continuous combined oestrogen/progestogen HRT regimens contraceptive?

It has been suggested that combinations of conjugated equine oestrogens 0.625 mg/day and norethisterone 0.7–1.05 mg/day (or medroxyprogesterone acetate 5 mg/day) taken together continuously may suppress ovulation. Confirmatory data from large-scale studies are lacking. Such combinations are associated with irregular vaginal bleeding in pre- and perimenopausal subjects and are not well tolerated. In addition, further work is required before such combinations can be recommended for general use outside research programmes since there are no adequate data on endometrial safety.

12.14 What about depot progestogens?

As stated elsewhere, oral progestogens can reduce the frequency and severity of vasomotor symptoms. It is likely that depot progestogen therapies have similar effects. However, the side-effects of depot progestogen regimens are well recognized. These include poorer cycle control and, in some women, weight gain and depression. One of the major disadvantages of depot progestogens is that treatment cannot be rapidly withdrawn should these problems occur. Many older women will, whilst using depot progestogen therapy, develop symptoms of oestrogen-deficiency. Oestrogen supplementation for symptom relief with concurrent use of depot progestogens may, in theory, lead to irregular vaginal bleeding.

12.15 What non-hormonal methods are available for the 'older' woman?

The following non-hormonal methods are available:

1. Sterilization
— male
— female

2. Intrauterine contraceptive device (IUCD)

3. Barrier methods
— condoms
— diaphragm/cervical cap/vault cap/vimule

4. Spermicides
— creams/jellies/foams/suppositories
— vaginal sponge
— C film

5. 'Natural' family planning.

They are comprehensively discussed in Guillebaud's *Contraception: Your Questions Answered* (see Guide to further reading). They will be only briefly referred to here.

12.16 How useful is the IUCD?

This may be particularly useful for an older woman, partly because of her own declining fertility (thus increasing the efficacy of the method) and also because there is a decreased risk of pelvic infection and expulsion of the device with increasing age. However, it is not appropriate for a woman with heavy periods or fibroids.

A woman may keep an IUCD in situ until 1 year after the menopause. It has been recommended that the device be removed at this time since postmenopausal cervical stenosis may make removal without anaesthetic impossible. The frequency with which this occurs in practice is not known.

12.17 Can 'natural' methods be used?

Since these methods depend on interpretation of various indices of fertility awareness, they may be unreliable in the older woman with menstrual irregularity and erratic ovulation.

12.18 What about the barrier methods and spermicides?

These are appropriate, and more reliable in the older age groups, because of decreased fertility and more proficient use. However, some couples seem reluctant to commence the use of these methods for the first time at this age, although this prejudice may stem from a lack of adequate education and counselling.

The use of spermicides alone can only be recommended for use after the age of 50 years and for the year following the menopause.

The contraceptive sponge is probably undervalued, but should be acceptable to many women over 45 years.

Appendix 1: Sample case history

Administrative details
Name, address, telephone number, date of birth

Attitudes/expectations to menopause and to HRT

Presenting complaints
- vasomotor
- sleeping pattern
- atrophic
- psychological
- collagen tissues

Include patient's interpretation of symptom pattern and its aetiology.
Note any previous self-medication for above symptoms.

Gynaecological history
Menstrual pattern, LMP, parity, current contraception, hysterectomy and/or oophorectomy (with reasons), smear result, fibroids, endometriosis, CIN, D&Cs, endometrial abnormality, PMS, dysmenorrhoea, etc.

Medical/surgical history
DVT, PE, MI, CVA, hypertension, diabetes, breast surgery and mammography, migraine, jaundice, gallstones, gastric surgery, colitis, epilepsy, fractures, otosclerosis, melanoma, thyroid disorder, steroid therapy, hypertriglyceridaemia, etc.

Current medication/allergies

Lifestyle
Marital status, employment, family, housing, smoking, alcohol, diet, exercise, stress, caffeine, etc.

Personal development history
Past psychiatric history, coping style, personality.

Current environment
Marital problems, financial problems, social supports, partner's adjustment, bereavement, divorce, separation, children leaving home, elderly parents, etc.

Family history
Breast cancer, osteoporosis, IHD/CVA, ovarian cancer.

Appendix 2: Useful addresses

The Amarant Trust
80 Lambeth Road
London SE1 7PW
Tel: (071) 401 3855
Fax: (071) 928 1702

British Menopause Society
83 High Street
Marlow
Buckinghamshire SL7 1AB
Tel: (0628) 890199

National Osteoporosis Society
PO Box 10
Barton Meade House
Radstock
Bath BA3 3YB
Tel: (0761) 32472

Women's Health Concern
83 Earls Court Road
London W8 6EF
Tel: (071) 938 3932

Women's Health Information Centre
52 Featherstone Street
London EC1Y 8RT
Tel: (071) 251 6580

Hysterectomy Support Network
3 Lynne Close
Green Street Green
Orpington
Kent BR6 6BS

Endometriosis Society
65 Holmdene Avenue
London SE24 9LD
Tel: (071) 737 0380

RELATE
76A New Cavendish Street
London W1
Tel: (071) 580 1087

Health Education Authority
Hamilton House
Mabledon Place
London WC1H 9TX

Family Planning Association
27-35 Mortimer Street
London W1N 7RJ
Tel: (071) 636 7866

Institute of Psychosexual Medicine
11 Chandos Street
London W1M 9DE
Tel: (071) 580 0631

National Association for the Childless
Birmingham Settlement
318 Summer Lane
Birmingham B19 3RL
Tel: (021) 359 4887

Women's National Cancer Control
Campaign
1 South Audley Street
London W1Y 5DQ
Tel: (071) 495 4995

British Association for Counselling
37a Sheep Street
Rugby
Warwickshire CV21 3BX
Tel: (0788) 78328

Guide to further reading

Chapter 1

Beaglehole R 1988 Oestrogen and cardiovascular disease. British Medical Journal 297: 571–572
Belchetz P 1989 Hormone replacement treatment — deserves wider use. British Medical Journal 298: 1467–1468
Purdie DW 1988 Broken bones — a gynaecological problem. British Journal of obstetrics and Gynaecology 95: 737–739
Stevenson JC 1990 Osteoporosis and cardiovascular disease in women: converging paths? Lancet 336: 1121–1122
Wells N 1987 Women's Health Today (No. 88). Office of Health Economics, London
Wilbush J 1988 Climacteric disorders — historical perspectives. In: Studd JWW, Whitehead MI (eds) The menopause. Blackwell Scientific, Oxford, pp 1–14

Chapter 2

Baird DT 1990 Biology of the menopause. In: Drife JO, Studd JWW (eds) HRT and osteoporosis. Springer-Verlag, London, pp 3–10
Belchetz P 1990 Endocrinology of the menopause. Practitioner 234: 491-493
Sherman BE 1987 Endocrinologic and menstrual alterations. In: Mishell DR (ed) Menopause: physiology and pharmacology. Year Book Medical, Chicago, pp 41–51

Chapters 3 and 4

Bourne T, Hillard TC, Whitehead MI et al 1990 Oestrogens, arterial status, and postmenopausal women. Lancet 335: 1470–1471
Brincat M, Studd J 1988 Skin and the menopause. In: Studd JWW, Whitehead MI (eds) The menopause. Blackwell Scientific, Oxford, pp 85–101
Bruce R, Stevenson JC 1990 Current understanding of osteoporosis. Comprehensive Therapy 16(9): 9–16
Bungay GT, Vessey MP, McPherson CK 1980 Study of symptoms in middle life with special reference to the menopause. British Medical Journal 281: 181–183
Campbell S, Whitehead MI 1977 Oestrogen therapy and the menopausal syndrome. Clinics in Obstetrics and Gynaecology 4. WB Saunders, London and Philadelphia, pp 31–47
Cardozo LD 1990 Oestrogen deficiency and the bladder. In: Drife JO, Studd JWW (eds) HRT and osteoporosis. Springer-Verlag, London, pp 57–68
Consensus Development Conference 1987 Prophylaxis and treatment of osteoporosis. British Medical Journal 295: 914–915
Crook D, Godsland IF, Wynn V 1988 Ovarian hormones and plasma lipoproteins. In: Studd JWW , Whitehead MI (eds) The menopause. Blackwell Scientific, Oxford, pp 169–181
Dennerstein L 1988 Psychiatric aspects of the climacteric. In: Studd JWW, Whitehead MI (eds). The menopause. Blackwell Scientific, Oxford, pp 43–54
Ettinger B 1987 Overview of the efficacy of hormonal replacement therapy. American Journal of Obstetrics and Gynecology 156: 1298–1303

Hunt K 1988 Perceived value of treatment among a group of long-term users of hormone replacement therapy. Journal of the Royal College of General Practitioners 38: 398–401

Hunter MS, Whitehead MI 1989 Psychological experience of the climacteric and postmenopause. Progress in Clinical and Biological Research 320: 211–224

Lobo RA 1990 Cardiovascular implications of estrogen replacement therapy. Obstetrics and Gynecology 75 (suppl 4): 18S–25S

Paganini-Hill A, Ross RK, Henderson BE 1988 Postmenopausal oestrogen treatment and stroke: a prospective study. British Medical Journal 297: 519–522

Ross RK, Pike MC, Mack TM, Henderson BE 1990 Oestrogen replacement treatment and cardiovascular disease. In: Drife JO, Studd JWW (eds) HRT and osteoporosis. Springer-Verlag, London, pp 209–222

Royal College of Physicians 1989 Fractured neck of femur — prevention and management. Royal College of Physicians, London

Stampfer MJ, Willett WC, Colditz GA et al 1985 A prospective study of postmenopausal estrogen therapy and coronary heart disease. New England Journal of Medicine 313: 1044–1049

Stevenson JC 1990 Pathogenesis, prevention and treatment of osteoporosis. Obstetrics and Gynecology 75 (suppl 4): 36S–41S

Vessey MP, Hunt K 1988 The menopause, hormone replacement therapy and cardiovascular disease: epidemiological aspects. In: Studd JWW, Whitehead MI (eds) The menopause. Blackwell Scientific, Oxford, pp 190–196

Whitehead MI 1985 The climacteric. In: Studd JWW (ed) Progress in obstetrics and gynecology. Volume 5. Churchill Livingstone, Edinburgh, pp 332–361

Whitehead MI 1987 The menopause. Practitioner 231: 37–42

Chapter 5

Editorial 1990 New treatments for osteoporosis. Lancet 335: 1065–1066

Siddle NC, Sarrell P, Whitehead MI 1987 The effect of hysterectomy on the age of ovarian failure: identification of a subgroup of women with premature loss of ovarian function and literature review. Fertility and Sterility 47: 94–100

Stevenson JC, Lees B, Devenport M et al 1989 Determinants of bone density in normal women: risk factors for future osteoporosis? British Medical Journal 298: 924–928

Studd JWW, Whitehead MI 1988 Selection of patients for treatment. Which therapy and for how long? In: Studd JWW, Whitehead MI (eds) The menopause. Blackwell Scientific, Oxford, pp 116–129

Chapter 6

Campbell S, Whitehead MI 1982 Potency and hepato-cellular effects of oestrogens after oral, percutaneous and subcutaneous administration. In: Van Keep PA, Utian W, Vermeulen A (eds). The controversial climacteric. MTP Press, Manchester, pp 103–125

Chetkowski RJ, Meldrum DR, Steingold KA et al 1986 Biologic effects of transdermal estradiol. New England Journal of Medicine 314: 1615–1620

Ganger K, Cust M, Whitehead MI 1989 Symptoms of oestrogen deficiency associated with supraphysiological plasma oestradiol concentrations in women with oestradiol implants. British Medical Journal 299: 601–602

Lane G, King R, Whitehead MI 1988 The effect of oestrogens and progestogens on endometrial biochemistry. In: Studd JWW, Whitehead MI (eds) The menopause. Blackwell Scientific, Oxford, pp 213–226

Lobo RA 1987 Absorption and metabolic effects of different types of oestrogens and progestogens. In: Gambrell RD (ed) Obstetrics and Gynecology Clinics of North America. WB Saunders, Philadelphia, 14(1): 143–168

Padwick ML, Endacott J, Whitehead MI 1985 Efficacy, acceptability and metabolic effects of transdermal oestradiol in the management of postmenopausal women. American Journal of Obstetrics and Gynecology 152: 1085–1089

Padwick ML, Pryse-Davies J, Whitehead MI 1986 A simple method for determining the optimal does of progestin in postmenopausal women receiving oestrogens. New England Journal of Medicine 315: 930–934

Whitehead MI, Siddle NK, Lane G et al 1986 The pharmacology of progestogens. In: Mishell DR (ed) Menopause: physiology and pharmacology. Year Book Medical, Chicago, pp 317–334

Whitehead MI, Hillard TC, Crook D 1990 The role and use of progestogens. Obstetrics and Gynecology 75 (suppl 4): 59S–79S

Chapter 7

Campbell S, Whitehead MI 1977 Oestrogen therapy and the menopausal syndrome. Clinics in Obstetrics and Gynecology 4. WB Saunders, London and Philadelphia, pp 31–47

Montgomery JC, Crook D 1990 Progestogens: symptomatic and metabolic side effects. In: Drife JO, Studd JWW (eds) HRT and osteoporosis. Springer-Verlag, London, pp 197–208

Siddle NC 1989 Psychological effects of different progestogens. In: Consensus Development Conference on Progestogens International Proceedings Journal 1: 214–217

Utian W 1978 Effect of postmenopausal estrogen therapy on diastolic blood pressure and body weight. Maturitas 1: 3

Chapter 8

Bergkvist L, Adami, Persson I et al 1989 Risks of breast cancer after estrogen and estrogen-progestin replacement. New England Journal of Medicine 321: 293–297

Boston Collaborative Drug Surveillance Program 1974 Surgically confirmed cases of gall bladder disease, venous thromboembolism, and breast tumours in relation to postmenopausal estrogen therapy. New England Journal of Medicine 290: 15–18

Brinton LA, Hoover RN, Fraumeni JF 1986 Menopausal oestrogens and breast cancer risk: an expanded case control study. British Journal of Cancer 54: 825–832

Brinton LA, Hoover RN, Szklo M et al 1981 Menopausal estrogen use and risk breast cancer. Cancer 47: 1417–1523

Buring JE, Hennekens CH, Lipnick RJ et al 1987 A prospective cohort study of postmenopausal hormone use and the risk of breast cancer in US women. American Journal of Epidemiology 125: 939–947

Colditz GA, Stampfer MJ, Willett WC, Hennekens CH, Rosner B, Speizer FE 1990 Prospective study of estrogen replacement therapy and risk of breast cancer in postmenopausal women. Journal of the American Medical Association 264: 2648–2653

Gambrell RD 1983 Breast disease in the postmenopausal years. Seminars in Reproductive Endocrinology 1: 27–40

Hiatt RA, Bawol R, Friedman GD, Hoover R 1984 Exogenous estrogen and breast cancer after bilateral oophorectomy. Cancer 54: 139–144

Hoover RN, Glass A, Finkle WD et al 1981 Conjugated estrogens and breast cancer risk in women. Journal of the National Cancer Institute 67: 815–820

Hoover RN, Gray LA, Cole P et al 1976 Menopausal estrogens and breast cancer. New England Journal of Medicine 295: 401–405

Hulka BS, Chambless LE, Deubner DC et al 1982 Breast cancer and estrogen replacement therapy. American Journal of Obstetrics and Gynecology 143: 638–644

Hunt K, Vessey M, McPherson K 1990 Mortality in a cohort of long-term users of hormone replacement therapy: an updated analysis. British Journal of Obstetrics and Gynecology 97: 1080–1086

Hunt K, Vessey M, McPherson, Coleman M 1987 Long-term surveillance of mortality and cancer incidence in women receiving hormone replacement therapy. British Journal of Obstetrics and Gynecology 94: 620–635

Jick H, Walker AM, Watkins RN et al 1980 Replacement estrogens and breast cancer. American Journal of Epidemiology 112: 586–594

Kaufman DW, Miller DR, Rosenburg L et al 1984 Non-contraceptive estrogen use and the risk of breast cancer. Journal of American Medical Association 252: 63–67

Kelsey JL, Fischer DB, Holford TR et al 1981 Exogenous estrogens and other factors in the epidemiology of breast cancer. Journal of the National Cancer Institute 67: 327–333

La Vecchia C, Decarli A, Parazzini F et al 1986 Non-contraceptive oestrogens and the risk of breast cancer in women. International Journal of Cancer 38: 853–858

McDonald I, Weiss N, Daling J et al 1986 Menopausal estrogen use and the risk of breast cancer. Breast Cancer Research and Treatment 7: 193–199

Mills PK, Beeson WL, Phillips RL, Fraser GE 1989 Prospective study of exogenous hormone use and breast cancer in Seventh Day Adventists. Cancer 64: 591–597

Nomura AM, Kolonel LN, Hirohata T et al 1986 The association of replacement estrogens with breast cancer. International Journal of Cancer 37: 45–53

Paginini-Hill A, Ross RK, Henderson BE 1989 Endometrial cancer and patterns of use of estrogen replacement therapy. British Journal of Cancer 59: 445–447

Persson I, Adami HO, Bergkvist L et al 1989 Risk of endometrial cancer after treatment with oestrogens alone or in conjunction with progestogens: results of a prospective study. British Medical Journal 298: 147–151

Ross RK, Paganini-Hill A, Gerkins VR et al 1980 A case-control study of menopausal estrogen therapy and breast cancer. Journal of the American Medical Association 243: 1635–1639

Sherman B, Wallace R, Bean J 1983 Estrogen use and breast cancer. Cancer 51: 1527–1531

Studd JWW, Magos A 1988 Oestrogen therapy and endometrial pathology. In: Studd JWW, Whitehead MI (eds) The menopause. Blackwell Scientific, Oxford, pp 197–212

Whitehead MI, Fraser D 1987 Controversies concerning the safety of estrogen replacement therapy. American Journal of Obstetrics and Gynecology 156: 1313–1322

Whitehead MI, Lobo RA 1988 Progestogen use in postmenopausal women. Lancet ii: 1243–1244

Wingo PA, Layde PM, Lee NC et al 1987 The risk of breast cancer in postmenopausal women who have used estrogen replacement therapy. Journal of the American Medical Association 257: 209–215

Chapters 9 and 10

Fraser D, Whitehead MI, Endacott J et al 1989 Are fixed-dose oestrogen/progestogen combinations ideal for all HRT users? British Journal of Obstetrics and Gynaecology 96: 776–782

Whitehead MI, Fraser D 1987 The effects of estrogens and progestogens on the endometrium: modern approach to treatment. In: Gambrell RD (ed) Obstetrics and Gynecology Clinics of North America. WB Saunders, Philadelphia 14(1): 299–320

Chapter 11

McEwan SR 1990 Prevention of cardiovascular disease in general practice. Horizons 4(4): 216–222

Mead M 1989 How to set up a health promotion clinic. Update 39: 847–854

Chapter 12

Guillebaud J 1985 Contraception for the older woman. In: Guillebaud J Contraception: your questions answered. Churchill Livingstone, Edinburgh, pp 286–291

Kubba A 1990 Contraception in the climacteric. In: Focus — the menopause. Medicom, London, pp 27–32

Upton V 1988 Contraception in the woman over forty. In: Studd JWW, Whitehead MI (eds) The menopause. Blackwell Scientific, Oxford, pp 289–304

Watson NR, Studd JWW, Riddle AI, Savvas M 1988 Suppression of ovulation by transdermal oestradiol patches. British Medical Journal 197: 900–901

Index